OXFORD MEDICAL PUBLICATIONS

New Brain Imaging Techniques and Psychopharmacology

BRITISH ASSOCIATION
FOR PSYCHOPHARMACOLOGY MONOGRAPHS

1. Psychopharmacology of affective disorders
   edited by E. S. Paykel and A. Coppen

2. Psychopharmacology of anticonvulsants
   edited by Merton Sandler

3. Psychopharmacology of old age
   edited by David Wheatley

4. Psychopharmacology and sexual disorders
   edited by David Wheatley

5. Psychopharmacology of the limbic system
   edited by Michael R. Trimble and E. Zarifian

6. Psychopharmacology: recent advances and future prospects
   edited by Susan D. Iversen

7. Psychopharmacology and food
   edited by Merton Sandler and Trevor Silverstone

8. Psychopharmacology and drug treatment of schizophrenia
   edited by P. B. Bradley and S. R. Hirsch

9. New brain imaging techniques and psychopharmacology
   edited by Michael R. Trimble.

New Brain Imaging Techniques and Psychopharmacology

BRITISH ASSOCIATION
FOR PSYCHOPHARMACOLOGY
MONOGRAPH
No. 9

EDITED BY

MICHAEL R. TRIMBLE
Consultant Physician in Psychological Medicine,
The National Hospitals for Nervous Diseases, London
Senior Lecturer in Behavioural Neurology
Institute of Neurology, London

Oxford New York Tokyo
OXFORD UNIVERSITY PRESS
1986

Oxford University Press, Walton Street, Oxford OX2 6DP
Oxford New York Toronto
Delhi Bombay Calcutta Madras Karachi
Kuala Lumpur Singapore Hong Kong Tokyo
Nairobi Dar es Salaam Cape Town
Melbourne Auckland

and associated companies in
Beirut Berlin Ibadan Nicosia

Oxford is a trade mark of Oxford University Press

Published in the United States
by Oxford University Press, New York

British Library Cataloguing in Publication Data
New brain imaging techniques and psychopharmacology.
—(British Association for psychopharmacology
monograph; no. 9)—(Oxford medical publications)
1. Brain—Diseases—Diagnosis   2. Diagnostic
imaging   3. Psychopharmacology
I. Trimble, Michael R.   II. Series
616.8′04754   RC386.6.R3
ISBN 0-19-261525-4

Library of Congress Cataloging in Publication Data
Main entry under title:
New brain imaging techniques and psychopharmacology.
(British Association for Psychopharmacology
monograph; no. 9) (Oxford medical publications)
Includes bibliographies and index
1. Diagnostic imaging—Congresses.   2. Brain—
Diseases—Diagnosis—Congresses.   3. Brain—Localization
of functions—Congresses.   4. Brain—Effect of drugs on—
Congresses.   5. Psychoses—Diagnosis—Congresses.
6. Psychopharmacology—Technique—Congresses.
I. Trimble, Michael R.   II. Series.   III. Series:
Oxford medical publications. [DNLM: 1. Brain—drug
effects.   2. Brain—radionuclide imaging.   3. Mental
Disorders—diagnosis.   4. Nuclear Magnetic Resonance.
5. Tomography, Emission Computed. W1 BR343D no.9/
WL 141 N5318]
RC386.6.D52N49   1986   616.8′04757   85–21528
ISBN 0-19-261525-4

Typeset by Joshua Associates Limited, Oxford
Printed in Great Britain by
St Edmundsbury Press
Bury St Edmunds, Suffolk

Preface

New methods of evaluating cerebral structure and function *in vivo* have been developed in recent years. The advent of CT scanning heralded a revolution in psychiatry, emphasizing once again the number of patients with psychiatric disability that have central nervous system changes which become identifiable with a relatively non-invasive radiological technique. In more recent years, other imaging methods have been developed, some of which are covered in this book, which will have great significance for psychopharmacology. The successful measurement of cerebral blood flow in the 1940s and 1950s was an important first step, being relatively inexpensive and easily repeatable. Chapter 8 emphasizes a recent study of cerebral blood flow in depression, the results of which may have bearing on the underlying pathogenesis of affective disorders.

With regards to psychopharmacology, the most important development has probably been positron emission tomography (PET). This method produces data on regional cerebral blood flow and metabolism in a variety of neuropsychiatric conditions, but because it primarily assesses function rather than structure it can be used to note changes in the former in relationship to disease states and treatment. The potential to radioactively label neurotransmitters and psychotropic drugs themselves is already with us, and in several chapters of this monograph the theory behind the technique, some of the data in psychiatric illness, and its future potential are discussed.

One of the latest additions to the techniques available is magnetic resonance imaging (MRI), formally referred to as nuclear magnetic resonance. Although completely in its infancy, the technique has enormous potential, and some preliminary data with regards to its use in neuropsychiatric illnesses are outlined.

Although some may consider it premature to attempt to bring together information in these fields, it is felt that knowledge about these techniques is limited, and their possible development not fully appreciated. It is hoped therefore that this book will prove a valuable early stepping stone to those interested in the use of imaging techniques in psychopharmacology, and that they will watch developments with great enthusiasm.

London   M.R.T.
February 1985

Contents

List of Contributors

J. D. BRODIE, Department of Psychiatry, New York University Medical Center, New York, NY 10016, USA.

M. S. BUCHSBAUM, Department of Psychiatry, University of California School of Medicine, Irvine, CA, USA.

G. M. BYDDER, Hammersmith Hospital, London, UK.

D. COMAR, Service Hospitalier Frédéric Joliot, CEA, Département de Biologie, 91406 Orsay, France.

T. J. CROW, Northwick Park Hospital, Watford Road, Harrow, Middlesex, UK.

L. E. DELISI, Clinical Neurogenetics Branch, NIH, NIMH, Bethesda, MD 20205, USA.

R. S. J. FRACKOWIAK, Hammersmith and National Hospitals, Royal Postgraduate Medical School and Institute of Neurology, London WC1, UK.

J. GIBBS, The National Hospital, Queen Square, London WC1, UK.

L. D. HALL, Department of Medicinal Chemistry, Cambridge University School of Clinical Medicine, Addenbrooke's Hospital, Cambridge CB2 2QQ, UK.

J. JACQUY, Department of Neurology, Hôpital Civil de Charleroi, Belgium.

E. C. JOHNSTONE, Northwick Park Hospital, Watford Road, Harrow, Middlesex, UK.

S. L. LUCK, Department of Chemistry, University of British Columbia, Vancouver, British Columbia, Canada V6T 1W5.

B. MAZIÈRE, Service Hospitalier Frédéric Joliot, CEA, Département de Biologie, 91406 Orsay, France.

M. MAZIÈRE, Service Hospitalier Frédéric Joliot, CEA, Département de Biologie, 91406 Orsay, France.

J. McCULLOCH, Wellcome Surgical Institute, University of Glasgow, Glasgow G61 1QH, Scotland, UK.

J. MENDLEWICZ, Department of Psychiatry, Hôpital Erasme, Free University of Brussels, Belgium.

T. NORWOOD, Department of Chemistry, University of British Columbia, Vancouver, British Columbia, Canada V6T IW5.

D. C. G. OWENS, Northwick Park Hospital, Watford Road, Harrow, Middlesex, UK.

V. RAJANAYAGAM, Department of Chemistry, University of British Columbia, Vancouver, British Columbia, Canada V6T IW5.

J. SCHACHTER, Department of Chemistry, University of British Columbia, Vancouver, British Columbia, Canada V6T IW5.

M. R. SMITH, Department of Psychiatry, New York University Medical Center, New York, NY 10016, USA.

R. E. STEINER, Hammersmith Hospital, London, UK.

M. R. TRIMBLE, Department of Psychological Medicine, National Hospitals, London WC1N 6BG, UKL.

P. UYTDENHOEF, Department of Neurology, Hôpital Civil de Charleroi, Belgium.

1

Mapping dynamic functional events in the central nervous system with 2-[^{14}C]deoxyglucose radioautography

JAMES McCULLOCH

INTRODUCTION

The advent of a range of quantitative radioautographic techniques for assessing various dynamic processes in the brain has provided neuroscientists with a novel approach with which to investigate functional events in the central nervous system. The dominant technique, in animal investigations, for functional mapping is the 2-[^{14}C]deoxyglucose technique for measuring local rates of glucose phosphorylation (Sokoloff *et al.* 1977). Conceptually and technically similar approaches for assessing local levels of blood flow (Sakurada *et al.* 1978) and local rates of protein synthesis (Smith *et al.* 1980) have also provided insight into functional processes but from a different perspective from that provided by the 2-deoxyglucose technique (see Kennedy *et al.* 1981; Collins and Nandi 1982; LeDoux *et al.* 1983; Freygang and Sokoloff 1958). Moreover, the availability of comparable techniques for investigating similar processes in man, in health and disease, has generated additional excitement in this area (see Phelps *et al.* 1982).

The present chapter will be devoted principally to the use of the 2-[^{14}C]deoxyglucose radioautographic technique in experimental animals. The extensive investigations in animals have been particularly instructive as to how 2-[^{14}C]deoxyglucose data (and other functional mapping material) should be interpreted if meaningful insight is to be gained from the clinical investigations of the function and dysfunction of the nervous system. Concepts rather than individual experimental series will be emphasized.

GLUCOSE UTILIZATION AS FUNCTIONAL ACTIVITY

Two simple principles provide the conceptual basis for the use of local rates of glucose utilization as an index of functional events in that region. Firstly, the energy requirements of cerebral tissue are derived almost exclusively from the aerobic catabolism of glucose (Sokoloff 1982; Siesjö 1978). Secondly, functional activity within any region of the central nervous system is intimately and directly related to energy consumption within that region (see Kennedy *et al.* 1975; Sokoloff 1982). Although statements such as these are often advanced, in many publications, as the sole justification for employing the radioautographic 2-deoxyglucose technique, the concept of 'functional activity' remains poorly defined. In this section glucose catabolism will be considered from neurochemical and neurophysiological viewpoints to clarify this concept of 'functional activity' which is central to all 2-deoxyglucose investigations and to relate it to other technical approaches.

Alternative routes of glucose catabolism

Glucose has a diverse involvement in intermediary metabolism quite distinct from its undisputed major role in energy generation. In the CNS, glucose is the principal source of carbon in lipids, as well as being the precursor of neurotransmitters such as GABA (γ-aminobutyric acid) and acetylcholine. A measurable proportion of glucose is metabolized via the pentose phosphate pathway, yielding not high-energy phosphates, but NADPH for the bio-synthesis of lipids and other macromolecules. A fraction of glucose carbon is incorporated into protein via the involvement of glucose in amino acid metabolism (for reviews see Maker *et al.* 1972 and Siesjö 1978). As the entry of the glucose carbon to these alternative metabolic pathways is subsequent to its phosphorylation, each will contribute to the rate of glucose utilization measured by the 2-deoxyglucose technique. It is fortunate that, under normal steady-state conditions, the proportion of glucose which is metabolized in the CNS via these possible routes is quantitatively small. For example, only about 2 per cent and 0.3 per cent of the entire cerebral glucose flux is directed toward lipid and protein synthesis, respectively (Maker *et al.* 1972). The contribution of the pentose phosphate pathway to the cerebral catabolism of glucose has proved extremely difficult to determine. The best estimates indicate that, in the rat, about 3 per cent of glucose is metabolized via this route (Siesjö 1978). The involvement of glucose as a precursor in the synthesis of acetylcholine and GABA is of particular interest for the 2-deoxyglucose technique in psycho-pharmacology. It has been estimated that, even at the maximum possible rate of synthesis of acetylcholine, only 1 per cent of the total pyruvate is required, the normal rate of synthesis being 10 per cent of its maximum level (Gibson *et al.* 1975). Thus, even large changes in the production of acetylcholine will con-tribute minimally to the measured rate of glucose use. Under normal condi-tions, a considerable fraction (approximately 8 per cent) of the total pyruvate passes via the 'GABA shunt', although this *per se* results in minimal loss to total energy generation from glucose provided the products of GABA catabolism (mainly succinate semialdehyde) are ultimately returned to the tricarboxylic acid cycle (Maker *et al.* 1972; Siesjö 1978).

Alternative energy-generating substrates to glucose

The energetic requirements of cerebral tissue are derived almost exclusively from the aerobic oxidation of glucose. Moreover, the brain possesses little flexibility in its choice of substrates *in vivo* (Sokoloff 1973, 1982; Siesjö 1978). Three possible modifications of the normal pattern of catabolism of glucose (namely, the accumulation of lactate, the utilization of glycogen and ketone bodies) must be considered because of their undoubted importance to the design and interpretation of 2-deoxyglucose experiments.

Anaerobic glycolysis generates a small fraction of the total ATP available compared to that for complete oxidative metabolism of glucose. Thus, under conditions in which the accumulation of lactate occurs, an elevated rate of glucose phosphorylation will be necessary to maintain an unchanged level of energy generation. Therefore, in experimentally induced seizures, in which focal accumulation of lactate is well recognized, the measured rates of glucose phosphorylation will no longer bear the same relationship to energy production which they do in normal animals. In contrast, neuropharmaco-logical manipulations are not normally associated with increased anaerobic glycolysis. For example, amphetamine, whose effects upon carbohydrate intermediary metabolism have been characterized in some detail, results in little net accumulation of lactate within brain tissue (see Siesjö 1978, for a more detailed discussion).

The oxidation of ketone bodies in the CNS represents one of the few energy-generating processes capable of replacing aerobic catabolism of glucose (Sokoloff 1973; Ruderman *et al.* 1974; Hawkins and Biebuyck 1979). In well-nourished animals, the levels of ketone bodies in arterial blood are extremely low (Ruderman *et al.* 1974; Gjedde and Crone 1975), and the contribution of ketone bodies to overall cerebral oxygen concentra-tion and energy metabolism is negligible (Hawkins *et al.* 1971; Ruderman *et al.* 1974). When the animals are deprived of food, arterial blood levels of ketone bodies rise rapidly (Ruderman *et al.* 1974; Gjedde and Crone 1975) and their rate of transfer across the blood–brain barrier is enhanced (Gjedde and Crone 1975) to such an extent that, after 24 h of starvation, the contribu-tion of ketone bodies to overall oxygen consumption has risen from less than 1 per cent to over 20 per cent (Ruderman *et al.* 1974). It is becoming increas-ingly apparent that the ability of different regions of the CNS to utilize ketone bodies displays marked heterogeneity, being far greater in the neocortex than in the caudate nucleus, for example (Hawkins and Biebuyck 1979). Although, these neurochemical data indicate that disruption of normal feeding should result in a heterogeneous alteration in regional glucose utiliza-tion, attempts to validate this experimentally have not been particularly suc-cessful. After 3 days of fasting, resulting in a marked hyperketonaemia, Corddry *et al.* (1982) did not observe any alterations in local rates of glucose phosphorylation, measured with the conventional [14]deoxyglucose tech-nique. While these latter data provide some reassurance, the practice of depriving subjects, human and animal, of food prior to 2-deoxyglucose studies must always be viewed with caution.

Physiological considerations

The 2-[14C]deoxyglucose radioautographic technique (Sokoloff *et al.* 1977) and its counterpart in humans, the [18F]deoxyglucose positron emission tomographic technique (Phelps *et al.* 1982: Chapter 2) provide only a measure of the rate at which glucose, delivered by the blood, is phosphorylated in a region of the CNS. The value of the rate of glucose phosphorylation results from its equivalence to the oxidative catabolism of glucose which is in turn indicative of energy generation. It is clearly important to consider the relative importance of the multitude of energy-demanding processes within the cell (transmitter synthesis, release, and reuptake; biosynthesis of macromolecules; ionic pumping etc.) and, additionally, the contribution which the various structural elements (such as neuronal perikarya and terminals, glia, axons, dendrites etc.) make to overall rates of glucose utilization. The information available at present is far from definitive despite its importance to the interpretation of all functional mapping investigations. It has been estimated that neurons are responsible for about 75 per cent of all oxygen consumed by the CNS (Siesjö 1978). The major portion of energy generated by the brain is used for ion transport, e.g. barbiturate anaesthesia producing an isoelectric EEG reduces oxidative catabolism of glucose to approximately 40 per cent of its normal level (Crane *et al.* 1978); even at this stage with electrocortical silence, glucose use can be reduced to approximately 20 per cent of the normal level by blocking Na^+–K^+ ATPase (adenosine triphosphatase) (Astrup *et al.* 1981). Thus almost 80 per cent of all energy generated may be destined for the maintenance of ionic gradients. The contribution of neuronal terminals to overall glucose utilization is likely to be considerably greater than that of neuronal perikarya as a direct consequence of the greater surface area to volume ratios in the neuronal terminals (Schwartz *et al.* 1979). In the superior cervical ganglion, glucose utilization correlates with the frequency with which the ganglion is stimulated orthodromically (Yarowski *et al.* 1983).

Although the diverse strands of evidence cited above indicate that *dynamic* alterations in glucose utilization reflects predominantly electrical activity in axonal terminals of neuronal pathways, it is important to recognize that increases and decreases in glucose use *cannot* be equated, merely, with neuronal excitation and inhibition respectively. Indeed, there is no basis for the idea that the energetic requirements of synaptic inhibition should be dissimilar to those associated with synaptic excitation, a view which has received substantial support from elegant investigations of long-term recurrent inhibition in the hippocampus (Ackermann *et al.* 1984).

The use of the 2-[^{14}C]deoxyglucose technique receives its most definitive support from the application of the technique itself in simple sensory stimulation and deprivation experiments. Deprivation of visual stimuli results in reductions in glucose utilization in neuroanatomical components of the visual system (i.e. dorsal lateral geniculate body, superficial layer of the superior colliculus and area 17 of the neocortex) whereas stimulation with diffuse light results in intensity-related increments in their glucose use (Figs. 1.1 and 1.2) (Kennedy *et al.* 1975; Miyaoka *et al.* 1979; McCulloch *et al.* 1980a; Toga and Collins 1981). Similarly, auditory stimulation or occlusion of the external auditory canals is associated with increases and

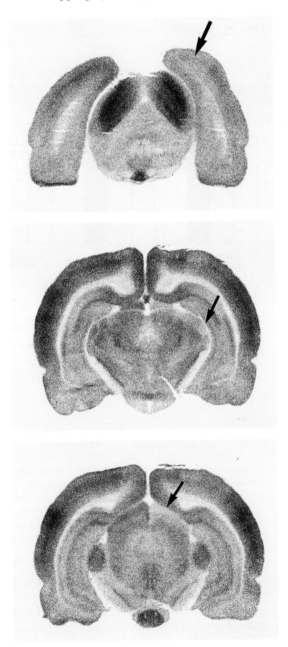

Fig. 1.1. Representative 2-deoxyglucose radioautograms of three primary visual areas in rats subjected to unilateral orbital enucleation. As the retinal pathway projects almost exclusively to the contralateral hemisphere in the rat, the asymmetrical optical density (and hence glucose use) in the visual cortex, lamina IV (top), lateral geniculate body (middle), and superficial layer of the superior colliculus (bottom) can be readily visualized.

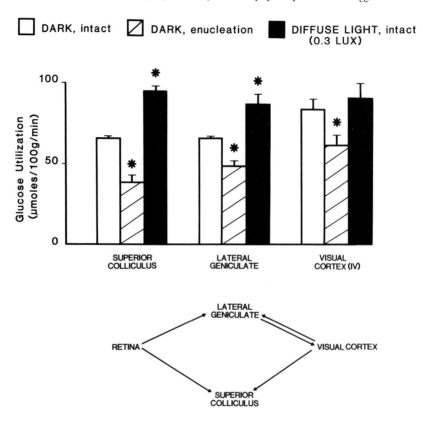

Fig. 1.2. Glucose utilization in primary visual areas during visual stimulation and deprivation. All animals were dark-adapted for 150 min prior to study. One group ('Dark, intact') possessed an intact visual system and were studied in the absence of detectable light. A second group ('Dark, enucleation') were subjected to orbital enucleation 4 h prior to being studied in the absence of detectable light; a third group ('Diffuse light, intact') possessed an intact visual system and were subjected to stimulation with diffuse light (0.3 lux, 1 Hz) during the measurement period. The anatomical arrangements within the visual system are depicted diagrammatically. Data are presented as means $\pm$ S.E.M. (*$P < 0.05$ from 'Dark, intact'). (From McCulloch *et al.* 1980a, and their unpublished observations.)

decreases in glucose utilization throughout the primary auditory pathway from the cochlear nucleus to auditory cortex (Sokoloff 1977; Sharp *et al.* 1981). Specific areas of enhanced glucose utilization can be demonstrated in specific areas of the olfactory bulb in response to stimulation with different odours (Sharp *et al.* 1975). Electrical stimulation of the sciatic nerve results in a marked increase in glucose use in the ipsilateral dorsal horn of the lumbar spinal cord corresponding directly to the local increase in neuronal activity (Kennedy *et al.* 1975). Further, enhanced glucose utilization in a discrete column of the somatosensory cortex of the rat resulting from the stimulation of a single whisker can be identified readily (Hand *et al.* 1978). Moderate hypotension provokes marked highly focal increases in glucose use in the areas of the brain known to be involved in the cardiovascular regulation (e.g. nucleus of the tractus solitarius, paraventricular and supraoptic nuclei of the hypothalamus etc.) (Savaki *et al.* 1982a). Thus, a correlation does appear to exist between the level of glucose utilization in neuroanatomical components of a functional system and the processing of information in that system.

METHODOLOGICAL DETAILS OF THE QUANTITATIVE RADIOAUTOGRAPHIC 2-[¹⁴C]DEOXYGLUCOSE TECHNIQUE

A detailed description of the theoretical basis and operational details for the use of 2-deoxyglucose in the determination of rates of local cerebral glucose utilization has been published (Sokoloff *et al.* 1977). Subsequently, a number of reviews have appeared in which various aspects of this particular method-ology and its application in neurobiology have been described (Sokoloff 1982; McCulloch 1982). The technique is designed to take advantage of the biochemical characteristics which result from the simple modification of the glucose molecule to deoxyglucose. The entry of glucose and 2-deoxyglucose into the CNS is mediated via the same carrier mechanism. In cerebral tissue, both glucose and 2-deoxyglucose are substrates for hexokinase which yields their respective hexose 6-phosphates. Although glucose 6-phosphate is metabolized subsequently (via the glycolytic and tricarboxylic acid pathways or the pentose phosphate pathway), 2-deoxyglucose 6-phosphate is not a substrate for glucose phosphate isomerase or glucose 6-phosphate de-hydrogenase, and its catabolism ceases at this point. Deoxyglucose 6-phosphate is a substrate for glucose 6-phosphatase (the action of which results in the hydrolysis of deoyglucose 6-phosphate to deoxyglucose), and the activity of this enzyme, if present in sufficient quantity, could seriously undermine the use of [¹⁴C]deoxyglucose in the determination of local cerebral glucose utilization (Hawkins and Miller 1978). In cerebral tissue glucose 6-phosphatase activity is extremely low (for references see Sokoloff *et al.* 1977; Sokoloff 1982).

Analysis of a model which describes the biochemical properties of glucose and deoxyglucose allows the rate of glucose utilization to be described mathematically by a single equation (the 'operational equation' of the tech-nique) (Sokoloff *et al.* 1977). The operational equation permits the local rate of glucose utilization to be calculated from (a) the levels of glucose and 2-[¹⁴C]deoxyglucose in plasma during the experimental period and (b) the total concentration of radioactivity within the region at the end of the experi-ment, provided the values of certain predetermined constants are known.

A full description of the operational details in their original and most definitive form has been published (Sokoloff *et al.* 1977). They can be summarized briefly. The measurement of local glucose utilization is initiated by the injection, via the venous catheter, of 2-[¹⁴C]deoxyglucose (125 μCi/kg). Fourteen timed samples of arterial plasma (approximately 40 μl) are obtained during the succeeding 45 min. The concentrations of glucose and

^{14}C in each of the samples is determined by automated enzymic assay and liquid scintillation counting, respectively. At approximately 45 min after the administration of the pulse of 2-deoxyglucose, the animal is sacrificed and the brain removed rapidly and frozen in an organic solvent (generally iso-pentane) which has been cooled between to -50 and $-70\,°$C. Sections (20 μm) are prepared in a cryostat at $-22\,°$C. Radioautograms are prepared from these sections by exposing them with medical X-ray film (such as Kodak SB-5) in light-tight X-ray cassettes for between 5 and 14 days. Local cerebral tissue concentrations of ^{14}C are determined by quantitative densitrometry, by reference to a number of [^{14}C]methylmethacrylate standards (generally about 10 different standards over a range 40–1200 nCi/g) which have been precalibrated for 20 μm brain sections of known concentrations. A set of these standards is exposed in each X-ray cassette along with the sections from the experimental animal.

A number of modifications can be made in the procedure without com-promising the reliability of the technique. For example, the radioautographic densitometric approach for quantifying ^{14}C concentrations in brain tissue can be substituted by dissection, either grossly or by the punch micro-dissection and liquid-scintillation counting. However, other seemingly simple modifications of the technique described by Sokoloff *et al.* (1977), some of which have found widespread use (most commonly, dispensing with the need for sampling arterial blood or performing only semiquantitative analysis of the radioautograms), do alter to varying degrees the accuracy and reliability of the technique (Kelly and McCulloch 1983a, b).

MERITS AND LIMITATIONS OF FUNCTIONAL MAPPING WITH 2-DEOXYGLUCOSE RADIOAUTOGRAPHY

In this section some of the advantages and disadvantages of deoxyglucose radioautography will be identified and illustrated by the use of specific examples. These features will also be emphasized in the following section when the application of the technique to neuropharmacology is considered.

Anaesthesia

In spite of the universally recognized effects of general anaesthetics upon almost every functional processes in the CNS, anaesthesia remains a necessary integral feature of many electrophysiological and neurochemical investigations. A major advantage of the 2-deoxyglucose technique is that it can be employed as readily in conscious animals as it can in anaesthetized animals. An excellent illustration of how a functional response in the CNS can be modified by anaesthesia are the studies of the effects of chloral hydrate (the anaesthetic most commonly employed in electrophysiology) upon the response of the substantia nigra to systemic administration of the dopamine agonist, apomorphine. In conscious rats, apomorphine adminis-tration *increases* glucose utilization in the pars compacta of the substantia nigra whereas in rats anaesthetized with chloral hydrate apomorphine

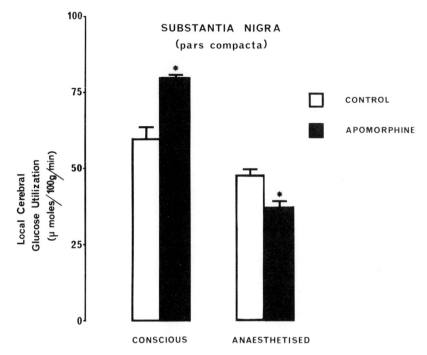

Fig. 1.3. Substantia nigra (pars compacta). Apomorphine (1 mg/kg, i.v.) *increases* glucose utilization in the region in fully conscious rats, whereas in animals anaesthetized with chloral hydrate, apomorphine *reduces* glucose use. Data are presented as means S.E.M. *$P < 0.05$ for the comparison between saline-treated control and apomorphine. (From Grome and McCulloch 1981.)

decreases glucose use in this key brain area (Fig. 1.3) (Grome and McCulloch 1981). These and other studies of anaesthetics with deoxyglucose radioautography (see also Grome and McCulloch 1983; Savaki *et al.* 1983) have produced a growing awareness of the importance of the choice of anaesthesia in investigations, electrophysiological or metabolic mapping, of basal ganglia function (see Waszczak *et al.* 1984).

Radioautography

The use of quantitative radioautography to measure local ^{14}C tissue concentrations is one of the attractive features of the original 2-deoxyglucose technique (Sokoloff *et al.* 1977). The spatial resolution with which functional events can be assessed with 2-^{14}C]deoxyglucose radioautography is immediately apparent from visual inspection of any radioautogram. The limit of spatial resolution with 2-^{14}C]deoxyglucose has been conservatively estimated at 100 μm across in sections 20 μm thick (Gochee *et al.* 1980), and, in practice, this allows glucose use to be easily assessed, for example, in the rat in single cortical layers (see Figs. 1.1 and 1.4), in individual hypothalamic nuclei, in small brain stem nuclei (locus coeruleus, dorsal raphe,

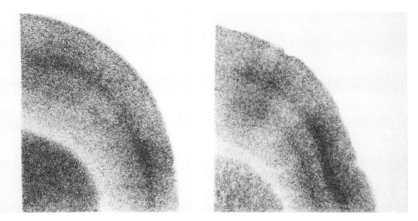

Fig. 1.4. Representative 2-deoxyglucose radioautograms of the rostral neocortex of the rat following saline (left) and apomorphine 1.5 mg/kg, i.v. (right) administration. The laminar activation (in layers IV and VI) produced by apomorphine with alternating columns of increased and decreased glucose use traversing the cortex can be identified readily. (From McCulloch *et al.* 1979.)

nucleus of tractus, solitarius etc.). The most important benefits which accrue from the use of quantitative data are not related simply to spatial resolution *per se* (the level of resolution is far inferior to single-cell recording or immunocytochemistry) but rather to the completeness and permanence of the map of functional events in that animal at the time of the experiment and particularly because it is not prejudiced in respect of regions to be investigated. As no *a priori* decision is required at the outset of the experiments as to which areas of the CNS are of interest in a particular study, 2-deoxyglucose radioautography can be most profitably employed in directing attention to areas whose involvement in a response is wholly unexpected. The investigations of dopaminergic influences upon cerebral cortical function are an excellent illustration of this feature (McCulloch *et al.* 1979). These investigations of the effects of the dopamine agonist, apomorphine, were designed to examine events in anterior cingulate cortex, one of the few areas of cortex in the rat which are known to contain specific dopaminergic receptors and nerve terminals. The radioautographic 2-deoxyglucose studies of the effects of systemically administered apomorphine confirmed that there were major functional changes in the anterior cingulate cortex, but in addition provided evidence that the influence of dopaminergic systems on cortical function extended beyond the known confines of the dopaminergic system, a finding not anticipated at the outset of the experiments (Figs. 1.4 and 1.5) (McCulloch *et al.* 1979). Apomorphine increased glucose use in specific areas of the dorsolateral rostral neocortex (an effect which can be blocked by low concentrations of haloperidol) in a highly neuroanatomically organized manner. The increases in glucose following apomorphine administration were columnar and confined to cortical layers IV and VI (Fig. 1.4).

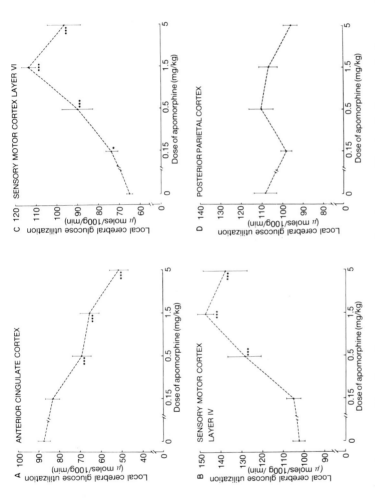

Fig. 1.5. Cerebral cortex and apomorphine. Log dose–response curves for glucose utilization in four cortical areas after the intravenous administration of apomorphine. Data are presented as means ± S.E.M. *$P < 0.05$, ***$P < 0.001$. Apomorphine significantly alters the rate of glucose use in areas containing dopaminergic receptors (e.g. anterior cingulate cortex) as well as in regions which do not contain dopaminergic receptors (e.g. sensory motor cortex). In the majority of cortical areas (e.g. posterior parietal cortex), apomorphine does not modify glucose utilization. (From McCulloch *et al.* 1979.)

The topography of these alterations in glucose use provided the clue to the interpretation of the observation for they corresponded almost exactly to the projection to the cortex arising in the ventral nucleus of the thalamus, which itself receives a major projection from the striatum via the globus pallidus. Thus, the dopaminergic system can modify events in the cerebral cortex either via receptor mechanisms intrinsic to the region (e.g. anterior cingulate cortex) or by altering activity via polysynaptic pathways in the non-dopaminergic thalamocortical systems (for more detailed discussions see McCulloch 1982). Moreover, these observations have enormous implications for the use of functional mapping techniques in man in clinical conditions, such as affective disorders, where dopaminergic dysfunction may be important.

Time constant

A major limitation of functional mapping with 2-[^{14}C]deoxyglucose is the long time period (generally 45 min) over which glucose utilization is calculated. Although this average glucose utilization is dominated by events in a 15-min period early in the investigation, the time course of 2-[^{14}C]deoxyglucose is inordinately long compared to that in electrophysiology for example. This limitation of the 2-deoxyglucose technique is a constraint resulting from the imprecision with which the kinetic rate constants for 2-deoxyglucose entry into and egress from the CNS are known for any condition (for discussion see Sokoloff 1982) and must be an inherent element in the design of any investigation. Radioautographic techniques for assessing local cerebral blood flow using freely diffusible isotopes in animals (Sakurada *et al.* 1978 as an example) have a shorter time constant (most commonly 30–60 s) than that for assessing local cerebral glucose utilization and, for this reason, have been proposed for mapping transient functional events in the CNS (LeDoux *et al.* 1983). As local levels of cerebral blood flow and glucose use are, normally, tightly coupled, the approach does possess some merits (Fig. 1.6) (McCulloch *et al.* 1982*a*)). However, it is one step further removed from cerebral 'function' with the potential for disruption of the flow–glucose use couple in 'abnormal' conditions (which can be as trivial as indomethacin treatment or hypercapnia or as gross as seizures or stroke). Moreover, because freely diffusible isotopes are employed, the spatial resolution of the cerebral blood flow radioautograms is poorer than those obtained in the measurement of glucose use; for example laminar variations in cortical blood flow cannot be discriminated with conventional [^{14}C]iodoantipyrine radioautography (Fig. 1.7).

APPLICATION OF FUNCTIONAL MAPPING WITH
2-DEOXYGLUCOSE TO NEUROPHARMACOLOGY

The primary aim in many neuropharmacological investigations which utilize the 2-deoxyglucose technique has been to characterize the functional consequences which are associated with manipulation for a particular neuro-

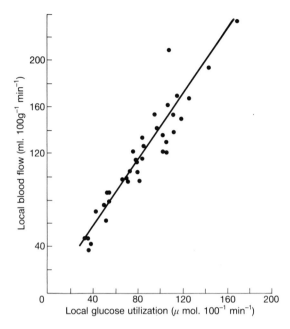

Fig. 1.6. The relationship between mean local cerebral blood flow and mean local cerebral glucose utilization in conscious rats. Each point represents data from one region of the CNS. There is an excellent correlation between local blood flow and local glucose use throughout the brain.

transmitter system (either by means of stereotactically placed lesions or stimulating electrodes or by the adminstration, systemically or intracerebrally, of putative receptor agonists and antagonists). There is already extensive literature dealing with the application of [14C]deoxyglucose radio-autography to neuropharmacology but, because of the constraints of space it could not be adequately covered in the present chapter. The present section will briefly summarize progress in areas relevant to psychopharmacology in man, and will provide references to key investigations in animals. A detailed review of the first 5 years of deoxyglucose radioautography in neuropharmacology is available elsewhere (McCulloch 1982).

Dopaminergic systems

Of all neurotransmitter systems in the CNS, dopaminergic systems have been the most extensively studied. From the earliest investigations of dopaminergic agonists and antagonists, it became clear that the regional distribution of alterations in glucose utilization resulting from a particular drug treatment *do not* correspond to the topography of the receptors for the drug in the CNS. If the analogy of the visual system is considered, the reason for this becomes immediately apparent; visual stimuli provoke alterations in glucose use not

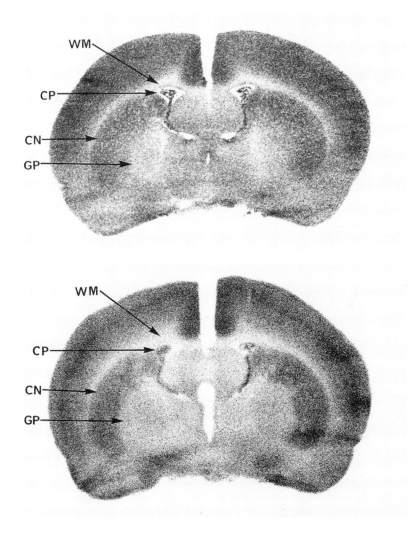

Fig. 1.7. Relative distribution of glucose utilization (left) and blood flow (right) at the level of the lateral ventricle. Local glucose utilization and local blood flow are proportional to the relative optical density of the region. WM, subcortical white matter; CP, choroid plexus of the lateral ventricle; CN, caudate nucleus; GP, globus pallidus.

only in the region which contains photoreceptors (i.e. the retina) but also in those regions which receive from the retina polysynaptic neuronal circuits in which the activity is regulated by the receptor (see Fig. 1.2). Thus, with the dopaminergic receptor agonist apomorphine the alterations in glucose utilization reflect metabolic events involved in the *initiation* of the central actions of apomorphine (in which dopaminergic receptors would be involved) as well as in the behavioural *expression* of the action of apomorphine (which would involve non-dopaminergic neural pathways as well as dopaminergic pathways). As alterations in motor function constitute a major element of the behavioural actions of apomorphine, it is hardly surprising that the administration of apomorphine results in alterations in glucose utilization in a large number of areas involved in motor control (cerebellum, red nucleus, ventral nucleus of the thalamus, subthalamic nucleus, inferior olivary nucleus, substantia nigra, globus pallidus, caudate nucleus) irrespective of the presence or absence of dopaminergic receptors (McCulloch *et al.* 1982b). The regional distribution of the changes in glucose use produced by amphetamine administration or by electrical stimulation of the ventral mesencephalon from where the principal dopaminergic systems arise is broadly similar to that produced by apomorphine (Wechsler *et al.* 1979; Orzi *et al.* 1983; Savaki *et al.* 1983; Esposito *et al.* 1984; Porrino *et al.* 1984). It must be emphasized that the disturbance in glucose utilization which results from activation of dopaminergic systems, whether pharmacological or electrical, is highly restricted in its distribution; in the vast majority of brain areas, glucose use is unaltered by enhanced dopaminergic activity (McCulloch *et al.* 1982b; Esposito *et al.* 1984). Moreover, the regions displaying alterations in glucose utilization are not randomly distributed, but part of neuroanatomically ordered circuits; for example, the globus pallidus, subthalamic nucleus, ventral thalamus, centromedial thalamus, lateral habenular nucleus, and raphe nuclei, all of which display alterations in glucose use with apomorphine, have major monosynaptic or polysynaptic connections with the caudate nucleus which, because of its abundance of dopaminergic receptors, is the most likely site for the initiation of the functional response to the drug. Stereotactic lesion and local intracerebral injection of dopamine experiments substantially confirm this view (Kelly and McCulloch 1982b; Brown and Wolfson 1983).

Although there is broad agreement concerning the regional distribution of the metabolic consequences of enhanced dopaminergic activity in extrapyramidal and motor areas, no coherent view has emerged of functional alterations in anatomical components of the limbic system. In general, metabolic alterations in the limbic system have been less marked and more difficult to detect following activation of dopaminergic systems than the local changes in areas involved in motor control. For example, although apomorphine significantly alters the rate of glucose utilization in anterior cingulate cortex, anterior thalamus, and some amygdaloid nuclei, the dopamine agonist fails to modify glucose use in a number of key areas of the limbic system, most notably the nucleus accumbens, septal nuclei, and entorhinal cortex, each of which contains dopamine receptors and is considered to be involved in the central actions of apomorphine (McCulloch *et al.* 1982b). These data emphasize one of the problems associated with the use of deoxyglucose radioautography in many areas of neurobiology—the apparently false negative observation. In the case of the nucleus accumbens and dopaminergic activation, the reason is far from clear at present; it may be related to limitation of the spatial resolution of the technique (with function-related alterations in energy production occurring below the threshold of detection) or subtle physiological factors (e.g. contingent intracranial self-stimulation of the ventral mesencephalon increases glucose use in the nucleus accumbens, whereas non-contingent experimenter-administered stimulation of the same location fails to alter glucose use in the nucleus accumbens (Porrino *et al.* 1984)).

In contrast to the well-developed hypotheses which have resulted from the use of dopaminergic agonists, no coherent understanding has yet emerged of the regional distribution of metabolic changes provoked by dopaminergic antagonists such as haloperidol (McCulloch *et al.* 1982*c*; Soncrant *et al.* 1984). This is particularly disappointing, for a clear view of cerebral metabolic actions of neuroleptics in animals would be of considerable value to investigators addressing the same problem in patients by employing positron emission tomography. In the rat, glucose use in the majority of brain areas is unaltered by haloperidol, except at very high concentrations (e.g. 10 mg/kg) where widespread reductions in glucose use are noted. At lower concentrations of haloperidol, which produce selective blockade of dopaminergic receptors, the alterations in glucose use are much more restricted in their distribution; in only three regions of the CNS (substantia nigra, pars compacta, lateral habenular nucleus, and nucleus accumbens, all of which play crucial roles in dopaminergic processes) was glucose use significantly elevated, whereas in a small number of major brain areas (neocortex, thalamic relay nuclei, the hippocampal formation) glucose use was depressed by haloperidol at concentrations which were without effect on the majority of areas studied (McCulloch *et al.* 1980*b*, 1982*c*).

There have been a number of investigations of the effects of chemical or electrolytic lesions of ascending dopaminergic systems. It now seems clear that if the substantia nigra, pars compacta, is *selectively* lesioned, the metabolic consquences are restricted to striatal efferent projections rather than the widespread depressions of forebrain glucose use which are asociated with non-selective large lesions placed in the central mesencephalon (see Wooten and Collins 1981).

Noradrenergic systems

The only major investigations of noradrenergic influences on local cerebral glucose utilization have been the examination of the functional consequences of the systemic administration of three putative α receptor antagonists; phentolamine, phenoxybenzamine, and yohimbine (Savaki *et al.* 1978, 1982*b*, *c*). The regional alterations fell into three general categories: (a) in a limited number of small nuclei, significant dose-related increases in glucose utilization were observed following administration of each of the α-blockers (e.g. the locus coeruleus, interstitial nucleus of the stria terminalis, para-ventricular and supraoptic nuclei, nucleus of the tractus solitarius, and dorsal motor nucleus of the vagus); (b) widespread reductions in glucose utilization were noted, particularly in neocortex and diencephanon; (c) glucose utilization in regions involved in the processing of auditory information displayed a different pattern of response from comparable areas involved in the processing of somatosensory or visual information (Savaki *et al.* 1978, 1982*a*, *b*). In contrast to dopaminergic systems, the intracerebral noradrenergic pathways are widely distributed throughout the CNS and, consequently, it has proven extremely difficult to resolve which metabolic alterations are associated with the initiation of the response from those involved in its expression. Investigation of the effects of unilateral lesion or stimulation of the locus coeruleus has been similarly fraught with difficulty (Abraham *et al.* 1979; Savaki *et al.* 1983, 1984).

The administration of the β-receptor antagonist, propranolol, leads to reductions in glucose utilization throughout almost the entire CNS, the reductions in the primary auditory areas being proportionately most marked. In only two regions of the CNS (the dentate gyrus and substantia nigra) was the level of glucose utilization maintained during propranolol administration (Savaki *et al.* 1978). As the authors themselves recognized, there are considerable doubts as to whether these reductions result from the selective blockade of central β-noradrenergic receptors in view of the enormous concentrations of propranolol administered (> 40 mg/kg, i.v.).

γ-Aminobutyric acid (GABA) systems

The intravenous administration of GABA receptor agonists, such as muscimol or THIP (4, 5, 6, 7 tetrahydoisoxayolo (4, 5, e-)pyridin-3-ol), results in reductions in glucose utilization throughout the entire CNS (Kelly and McCulloch 1982; Palacios *et al.* 1982), presumably reflecting the widespread distribution of GABA receptors and their involvement in almost every functional process. Although glucose use in every area of the CNS could be reduced by muscimol and THIP, examination of the log dose–response curves provides unequivocable evidence of regional heterogeneity of the susceptibility of glucose use to be modified by both muscimol and THIP. The regions in which glucose utilization was extremely sensitive to change, displaying reductions of approximately 40 per cent following muscimol (1.5 mg/kg) or THIP (10 mg/kg) administration, included all layers of the neocortex (frontal, sensory motor, posterior parietal, primary auditory, and visual cortices), the lateral portion of the caudate nucleus, and some thalamic nuclei (lateral geniculate body, mediodorsal and ventrolateral nuclei). Regions displaying more modest reductions in glucose utilization, approximately 20 per cent following muscimol (1.5 mg/kg) and THIP (10 mg/kg) administration, included most extrapyramidal regions (substantia nigra, pars compacta and reticulata, globus pallidus, subthalamic nucleus, medial portion of the caudate nucleus) a number of cortical and subcortical limbic areas (cingulate and olfactory cortices, hippocampus, nucleus accumbens, anterior thalamus), and medial raphe nucleus. In contrast, in a

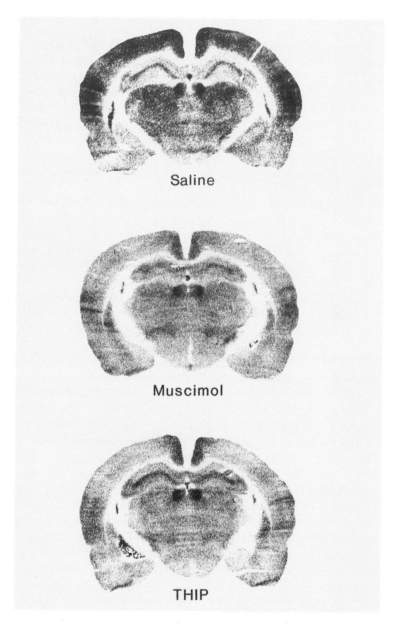

Saline

Muscimol

THIP

Fig. 1.8. GABAergic agonists, muscimol and THIP, and local glucose utilization. Representative deoxyglucose radioautograms at the level of the thalamus. Saline-treated control (top); optical density in the cerebral cortex, thalamus, and lateral habenula (epithalamus) are similar. Following muscimol (1.5 mg/kg, i.v.) (middle) or THIP (10 mg/kg, i.v.) (bottom), optical density in the thalamus and cortex are markedly reduced relative to the lateral habenula in which glucose use is unaltered by these agents. (Data from Kelly and McCulloch 1982a.)

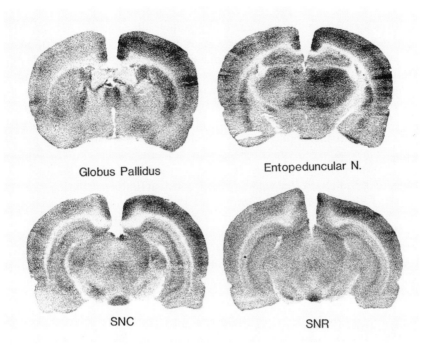

Globus Pallidus

Entopeduncular N.

SNC

SNR

Fig. 1.9. Intrastriatal injection of the GABAergic agonist, muscimol. 2-Deoxyglucose radioautograms from representative animals receiving muscimol (500 ng) at four coronal levels of the CNS. Ipsilateral areas are on the left. Asymmetries in optical density reflect asymmetries of glucose utilization. At the level of the globus pallidus (upper left) the marked ipsilateral reductions (relative to the contralateral hemisphere) in the cortex and caudal portion of the caudate nucleus, and the increased glucose utilization in the globus pallidus, can be readily seen. At the level of the entopeduncular nucleus (upper right) the increased glucose use ipsilateral in this nucleus and decreased use in the ventral thalamic nucleus can be discerned. At the level of the substantia nigra (both lower figs.) the increases in glucose use in the ipsilateral pars compacta (SNC) and pars reticulata (SNR), particularly in the most ventral aspect, are visible in the radioautograms. (From Kelly and McCulloch 1984.)

large number of regions (including cerebellum and related nuclei such as the inferior olivary, red and vestibular nuclei, white matter, pontine reticular formation, hypothalamus, lateral habenula and amygdala), there were only minimal (approximately 10 per cent) reductions in glucose utilization following muscimol (1.5 mg/kg) and THIP (10 mg/kg) administration (see Figs. 1.8 and 1.9). The regional distribution of alterations in glucose utilization following muscimol and THIP administration, which does not correspond to the known topography of GABAergic neurons and receptors, reflects rather the integrated overall consequences of enhanced GABAergic activity (Kelly and McCulloch 1982; Palacios *et al.* 1982).

A number of studies have explored the functional consequences of administering the GABAergic antagonist, bicuculline (see Ben-Ari *et al.*

1981; Palacios *et al.* 1982). Although there is general agreement that this convulsant can provide spectacular radioautographic images, there are wide differences among the various experimenter groups in their descriptions of the topography of the alterations in glucose utilization, presumably reflecting differences in the intensity of the seizure provoked by bicuculline and its temporal progresion. Moreover, there has been little discussion in the deoxyglucose studies of the role local GABAergic mechanisms play in producing the disordered patterns of cerebral glucose use. A further difficulty with the application of the deoxyglucose technique to the bicuculline response involves changes in numerical values of the lumped constant and kinetic rate constants used in the calculation of local rates of glucose utilization. As the values of these constants influence the local uptake of 2-[^{14}C]deoxyglucose visualized in the radioautograms, quantification of absolute rates of glucose utilization in seizures is fraught with difficulty.

One conceptually important feature to emerge from the investigations of GABAergic pharmacology has been the recognition of the marked differences in the patterns of altered glucose use which result from a discrete, local activation of GABAergic mechanisms compared to that produced by systemic administration.

CONCLUDING COMMENTS

The radioautographic 2-deoxyglucose technique has, in the few years since its development, found wide acceptance in almost all neuroscientific disciplines. It is disappointing that such detailed consideration must still be given to neurochemical and methodological aspects which are fundamental to accurate application of the technique. Until very recently, the interpretation of neuropharmacological investigations utilizing the radioautographic deoxyglucose or its PET counterparts in man has often been poorly developed, the presentation of observations in many of the earlier investigations being merely phenomenological.

Appreciation of functional mapping data has been enhanced by considering *not* simply the anatomical distribution of receptors, but rather by considering the receptor topography in conjunction with the neuroanatomical circuits in which the receptors regulate the activity. There is now overwhelming evidence that this must be the basis for providing rational interpretation of the regional patterns of disordered glucose utilization (or other dynamic techniques) which are observed in functional mapping in animals and in man. With this perspective, functional mapping will progress from identifying *where* events are occurring in the CNS to establishing *why* they occur in that particular region.

REFERENCES

Abraham, W. C., Delanoy, R. L., Dunn, A. J., and Zornetzer, S. F. (1979). Locus coeruleus stimulation decreases deoxyglucose uptake in ipsilateral mouse cerebral cortex. *Brain Res.* **172**, 387–92.

Ackermann, R., F., Finch, D. M., Babb, T. L., and Engle, J., Jr. (1984). Increased glucose metabolism during long-duration recurrent inhibition of hippocampal pyramidal cells. *J. Neurosci.* **4(1)**, 251–64.

Astrup, J., Sørensen, P. M., and Sørensen, H. R. (1981). Oxygen and glucose consumption related to $Na^+–K^+$ transport in canine brain. *Stroke* **12**, 726–30.

Ben-Ari, Y., Tremblay, E., Riche, D., Ghilini, G., and Naquet, R. (1981). Electrographic, clinical and pathological alterations following systemic administration of kainic acid, bicuculline or pentetrazole: metabolic mapping using the deoxyglucose method with special reference to the pathology of epilepsy. *Neuroscience* **6**, 1361–91.

Brown, L. L. and Wolfson, L. I. (1983). A dopamine-sensitive striatal efferent system mapped with [^{14}C]deoxyglucose in the rat. *Brain Res.* **261**, 213–29.

Collins, R. C. and Nandi, N. (1982). Focal seizures disrupt synthesis in seizure pathways: An autoradiographic study using L-[^{14}C]leucine. *Brain Res.* **248**, 109–19.

Corddry, D. H., Rapoport, S. I., and London, E. D. (1982). No effect of hyperketonemia on local cerebral glucose utilization in conscious rats. *J. Neurochem.* **38**, 1637–41.

Crone, P. D., Braun, L. D., Cornford, E. M., Cremer, J. E., Glass, J. M., and Oldendorf, W. H. (1978). Dose dependent reduction of glucose utilization by pentobarbital in rat brain. *Stroke* **9**, 12–18.

Esposito, R. U., Porrino, L. J., Seeger, T. F., Crane, A. M., Everist, H. D., and Pert, A. (1984). Changes in local cerebral glucose utilization during rewarding brain stimulation. *Proc. Natl. Acad. Sci. USA* **81**, 635–9.

Freygang, W. H., Jr. and Sokoloff, L. (1958). Quantitative measurement of regional circulation in the central nervous system by the use of radioactive inert gas. *Adv. Biol. Med. Phys.* **6**, 263–79.

Gibson, G. E., Jope, R., and Blass, J. P. (1975). Decreased synthesis of acetylcholine acompanying impaired oxidation of pyruvic acid in rat brain slices. *Biochem. J.* **148**, 17–23.

Gjedde, A. and Croue, C. (1975). Induction process in blood brain transfer of ketone bodies during starvation. *Am. J. Physiol.* **229**, 1165–9.

Goochee, C., Rasband, W., and Sokoloff, L. (1980). Computerized densitometry and color coding of [14C]deoxyglucose autoradiographs. *Ann. Neurol.* **7**, 359–70.

Grome, J. J. and McCulloch, J. (1981). The effects of chloral hydrate anesthesia on the metabolic response in the substantia nigra to apomorphine. *Brain Res.* **214**, 223–8.

—— and McCulloch, J. (1983). The effects of apomorphine upon local cerebral glucose utilization in conscious rats and in rats anesthetized with chloral hydrate. *J. Neurochem.* **40**, 567–76.

Hand, P. J., Greenberg, J. H., Miselis, R. R., Weller, W. L., and Reivich, M. (1978). A normal and altered cortical column: a quantitative and qualitative [^{14}C]2-deoxyglucose study. *Neurosci. Abs.* **4**, 553.

Hawkins, R. A. and Biebuyck, J. F. (1979). Ketone bodies are selectively used by individual brain regions. *Science* **205**, 325–7.

—— and Miller, A. L. (1978). Loss of radioactive 2-deoxy-α-glucose-6-phosphate from brains of conscious rats: implications for quantitative autoradiographic determination of regional glucose utilization. *Neuroscience* **3**, 251–8.

—— Williamson, D. H. and Krebs, A. H. (1971). Ketone body utilization by adult and suckling rat brain *in vivo*. *Biochem. J.* **122**, 13–18.

Kelly, P. A. T. and McCulloch, J. (1982a). Effects of the putative GABAergic agonists, muscimol and THIP, upon local cerebral glucose utilisation. *J. Neurochem.* **39**, 613–24.

—— and —— (1982b). GABAergic and dopaminergic influences on glucose utilization in the extrapyramidal system. *Brit. J. Pharmac.* **76**, 209P.

Kelly, P. A. T. and McCulloch, J. (1983a). A critical appraisal of semiquantitative analysis of 2-deoxyglucose autoradiograms. *Brain Res.* **269**, 165–7.

—— and —— (1983b). A potential error in modifications of the [¹⁴C]2-deoxyglucose technique. *Brain Res.* **260**, 182–7.

—— and —— (1984). Extrastriatal circuits activated by intrastriatal muscimol: a ¹⁴C-2-deoxyglucose investigation *Brain Res.* **292**, 357–66.

Kennedy, C., Des Rosiers, M. H., Jehle, J. W., Reivich, M., Sharpe, F., and Sokoloff, L. (1975). Mapping of functional neural pathways by autoradiographic survey of local metabolic rate with [¹⁴C]deoxyglucose. *Science* **187**, 850–3.

—— Suda, S., Smith, C. B., Miyaoka, M., Ito, M., and Sokoloff, L. (1981). Changes in protein synthesis underlying functional plasticity in immature monkey visual system. *Proc. Natl. Acad. Sci. USA* **78**, 3950–3.

LeDoux, J. E., Thompson, M. E., Iadecola, C., Tucker, L. W., and Reis, D. J. (1983). Local cerebral blood flow increases during auditory and emotional processing in the conscious rat. *Science* **221**, 576–8.

Maker, H. S., Clarke, D. D., and Lajtha, A. L. (1972). Intermediary metabolism of carbohydrates and amino acids. In *Basic Neurochemistry* (eds. G. J. Seigel, R. W. Albers, R. Katzman, and B. W. Lagranoff) pp. 279–307. Little, Brown & Co., Waltham, MA.

McCulloch, J. (1982). Mapping functional alterations in the CNS with [¹⁴C]–deoxyglucose. In *Handbook of psychopharmacology* (eds. L. L. Iversen, S. D. Iversen, and S. H. Snyder) Vol. 15, pp. 321–410. Plenum, New York.

—— Kelly, P. A. T. and Ford, I. (1982a). Effect of apomorphine on the relationship between local cerebral glucose utilization and local cerebral blood flow (with an appendix on its statistical analysis). *J. Cerebr. Blood Flow Metabol.* **2**, 487–99.

—— Savaki, H. E., and Sokoloff, L. (1980b). Influence of dopaminergic systems on the lateral habenular nucleus of the rat. *Brain Res.* **194**, 117–24.

—— —— and —— (1982a). Distribution of effects of haloperidol on energy metabolism, in the rat brain. *Brain Res.* **243**, 81–90.

—— —— —— McCulloch, M. C., and Sokoloff, L. (1979). Specific distribution of metabolic alterations in cerebral cortex following apomorphine administration. *Nature, Lond.* **282**, 303–5.

—— —— —— and —— (1980b). Retina-dependent activation by apomorphine of metabolic activity in the superficial layer of the superior colliculus. *Science* **207**, 313–15.

—— —— —— Jehle, J., and Sokoloff, L. (1982b). The distribution of alterations in energy metabolism in the rat brain produced by apomorphine. *Brain Res.* **243**, 67–80.

Miyaoka, M., Shinohara, M., Batipps, M., Pettigrew, K. D., Kennedy, C., and Sokoloff, L. (1979). The relationship between the intensity of the stimulus and the metabolic response in the visual system of the rat. *Acta Neurol. Scand.* **60, Suppl. 72**, 16–17.

Orzi, F., Dow-Edwards, D., Jehle, J., Kennedy, C., and Sokoloff, L. (1983). Comparative effects of acute and chronic administration of amphetamine on local cerebral glucose utilization in the conscious rat. *J. Cereb. Blood Flow Metab.* **3**, 154–60.

Palacios, J. M., Kuhar, M. J., Rapoport, S. I., and London, E. D. (1982). Effects of γ-aminobutyric acid agonist and antagonist drugs on local cerebral glucose utilization. *J. Neurosci.* **2**, 853–60.

Phelps, M. E., Mazziotta, J. C., and Huang, S.-C. (1982). Study of cerebral function with positron computed tomography. *J. Cereb. Blood Flow Metab.* **2**, 113–62.

Porrino, L. J., Esposito, R. U., Seeger, T. F., Crane, A. M., Pert, A., and Sokoloff, L. (1984). Metabolic mapping of the brain during rewarding self-stimulation. *Science* **224**, 306–9.

Ruderman, N. B., Ross, P. S., Berger, M., and Goodman, M. N. (1974). Regulation of glucose and ketone-body metabolism in brain of anaesthetized rats. *Biochem. J.* **138**, 1–10.

Sakurada, O., Kennedy, C., Jehle, J., Brown, J. D., Carbin, G. L., and Sokoloff, L. (1978). Measurement of local cerebral blood flow with iodo[^{14}C]antipyrine. *Am. J. Physiol.* **234**, H59–H66.

Savaki, H. E., Graham, D. I., and McCulloch, J. (1982a) Differential effects of locus coeruleus lesions upon metabolic activity in CNS nuclei involved in cardiovascular regulation. *Brain Res.* **271**, 109–14.

—— Macpherson, H., and McCulloch, J. (1982b). Alterations in local cerebral glucose utilization during hemorrhagic hypotension in the rat. *Circ. Res.* **50**, 633–4.

—— Desban, M., Glowinski, J., and Besson, M.-J. (1983). Local cerebral glucose consumption in the rat. II. Effects of unilateral substantia nigra stimulation in conscious and in halothane-anesthetized animals. *J. Comp. Neurol.* **213**, 46–65.

—— Graham, D. I., Grome, J. J., and McCulloch, J. (1984). Functional consequences of unilateral lesion of the locus coeruleus: A quantitative [^{14}C]2-deoxyglucose investigation. *Brain Res.* **292**, 239–49.

—— Kadekaro, M., Jehle, J., and Sokoloff, L. (1978). α- and β-adrenoreceptor blockers have opposite effects on energy metabolism of the central auditory system. *Nature, Lond.* **276**, 521–3.

—— McCulloch, J., and Sokoloff, L. (1982a). The central noradrenergic system in the rat: metabolic mapping with α-adrenergic blocking agents. *Brain Res.* **234**, 65–79.

—— McCulloch, J., Kadekaro, M., and Sokoloff, L. (1982c). Influence of α-receptor blocking agents upon metabolic activity in nuclei involved in central control of blood pressure. *Brain Res.* **233**, 347–58.

Schwartz, W. J., Smith, C. B., Davidsen, L., Savaki, H., Sokoloff, L., Mata, M., Fink, D. J., and Gainer, H. (1979). Metabolic mapping of functional activity in the hypothalamo-neurohypophysial system of the rat. *Science* **205**, 723–5.

Sharp, F. R., Kauer, J. S., and Shepherd, G. M. (1975). Local sites of activity-related glucose metabolism in rat olfactory bulb during olfactory stimulation. *Brain Res.* **98**, 596–600.

—— Ryan, A. F., Goodwin, P., and Woolf, N. K. (1982). Increasing intensities of wide band noise increase [^{124}C]2-deoxyglucose uptake in gerbil central auditory structures. *Brain Res.* **230**, 87–96.

Siesjö, B. K. (1978). *Brain Energy Metabolism.* Wiley, New York.

Smith, C. B., Davidsen, L., Deibler, G., Patlak, C., Pettigrew, K., and Sokoloff, L. (1980). A method for determination of local rates of protein synthesis in brain. *Trans. Am. Soc. Neurochem.* **11**, 94.

Sokoloff, L. (1973). Metabolism of ketone bodies by the brain. *Ann. Rev. Med.* **23**, 271–80.

—— (1977). Relation between physiological function and energy metabolism in the central nervous system. *J. Neurochem.* **29**, 13–26.

—— (1982). The radioactive deoxyglucose method. Theory, procedure, and applications for the measurement of local glucose utilization in the central nervous system. In *Advances in neurochemistry*. (eds. B. W. Agranoff and M. H. Aprison) Vol. 4, pp. 1–82. Plenum, New York.

—— Reivich, M., Kennedy, C., Des Rosiers, M. H., Patlak, C. S., Pettigrew, K. D., Sakurada, O., and Shinohara, M. (1977). The [^{14}C]deoxyglucose method for the measurement of local cerebral glucose utilization: theory, procedure, and normal values in the conscious and anesthetized albino rat. *J. Neurochem.* **28**, 897–917.

Toga, A. W. and Collins, R. C. (1981). Metabolic response of optic centers to visual stimuli in the albino rat: anatomical and physiological considerations. *J. Comp. Neurol.* **199**, 443–64.

Waszczak, B. L., Lee, E. K., Ferraro, T., Hare, T. A., and Walters, J. R. (1984). Single unit responses of substantia nigra pars reticulata neurons to apomorphine: effects of striatal lesions and anesthesia. *Brain Res.* **306** , 307–18.

Wechsler, L. R., Savaki, H. E., and Sokoloff, L. (1979). Effects of *d*- and *l*-amphetamine on local cerebral glucose utilization in the conscious rat. *J. Neurochem.* **32** , 15N22.

Wooten, G. F. and Collins, R. C. (1981). Metabolic effects of unilateral lesion of the substantia nigra. *J. Neurosci.* **1** , 281–91.

Yarowski, P., Kadekaro, M., and Sokoloff, L. (1983). Frequency-dependent activation of glucose utilization in the superior cervical ganglion by electrical stimulation of cervical sympathetic trunk. *Proc. Natl. Acad. Sci. USA* **80** , 4179–83.

2

An introduction to positron tomography and its application to clinical investigation

RICHARD S. J. FRACKOWIAK

Positron tomography is a technique for measuring tissue radioisotope concentrations regionally in the live intact subject. It has exquisite sensitivity, being capable of detecting and quantifying picomolar concentrations in samples of tissue of $1-3$ cm^3. It has the further advantage of being able to make the measurements in any region of the tissue or body of interest by using tomographic techniques. The measurements derived from deep structures remain accurate despite the fact that they are all made non-invasively with external detectors.

In this chapter the principles underlying measurement of isotope concentrations with positron tomography (PET) are set out, and then the way this capability is used to study cerebral function in man is described. This will involve a short description of tracer techniques, their formulation, verification, and application. Finally, an attempt to foresee how this method of investigating the human brain *in vivo* might be applicable to psychiatric disease will be made. This chapter should also serve as an introduction to the remaining chapters in this monograph which relate to PET studies in neuropsychiatric disorders.

IMAGING AND MEASUREMENT

PET is usually thought of as an imaging method. This has caused considerable confusion, as direct comparisons are immediately made with other cerebral imaging techniques such as magnetic resonance imaging (NMR), X-ray CT scanning and single photon emission tomogrpahy (SPECT). This confusion extends to concepts regarding the interpretation of PET data and indications for PET investigation. NMR and CT scanning provide tomographic images of cerebral structure, the one as a distribution of the density of protons constituting the brain substance and the other a distribution of X-ray-stopping power, also a function of density. PET in contrast provides metabolic or functional information and intrinsically little or no structural data. Functional information is communicated very approximately by images and requires quantification to be meaningful. Thus the imaging capabilities of PET, which derive from the mode of data collection, can at best serve as an aide memoire, or illustration, of much more detailed data pertaining to a variety of cerebral functions.

Potentially the processes that can be studied with PET are legion and limited only by considerations of appropriate tracer design and the ability to describe the temporal and spatial fate of an injected tracer in terms of a metabolic or physiological process. This in turn depends on the ability of the tomograph to make the desired measurements with the correct degree of spatial and temporal resolution. Thus, as will be described below, well validated and established techniques exist for measuring cerebral blood flow (CBF), blood volume (CBV), oxygen and glucose consumption (CMRO$_2$ and CMRGlc), fractional oxygen and glucose extractions (OER, GER), the stoichiochemistry of oxidative metabolism of glucose (MR), and regional haematocrit. Measurement of cerebral protein metabolism, pH, and permeability characteristics of the blood–brain barrier are all in advanced stages of development. The most recent and exciting techniques are the advances in measuring presynaptic vesicular uptake of L-dopa, its storage capacity and possible turnover, as well as dopamine receptor binding characteristics and distributions.

It is clear that each technique using PET requires a number of developmental steps before it becomes established. A radiochemical synthesis of a suitably labelled tracer which will have the correct biological characteristics is required. A biochemical and physiological description of the sites of distribution and pathways and sites of metabolism following introduction into the body by various routes must be obtained. The necessary tissue and blood or plasma measurements must be defined as well as the need for equilibrium or time course data. The variable of interest must be describable mathematically in terms of the measurements which can be made. Finally, normal data must be established in the human so that disturbances due to disease or therapeutic intervention can be assessed.

INSTRUMENTATION

The power of PET lies in its capacity to quantify tracer concentrations in absolute units. This means that the measurement of the physiological or other variable can be expressed in absolute terms, so that measurements made within patient groups or within individuals before and after intervention, or with the passage of time, are all strictly comparable. This capability is not available to SPECT. It is a function of the decay of isotopes by positron emission and a specific form of detecting the resulting radiation known as annihiliation coincidence detection.

Positrons emitted from decaying nuclei are in effect positively charged electrons which, within a very short distance of their parent nucleus, meet an electron and interact giving rise to an annihilation reaction. This converts the mass of the two particles into two oppositely directed monoenergetic gamma rays (511 KeV). If unhindered, these rays, which move at the speed of light, can be detected by crystals placed 180° apart to either side of the disintegrating nucleus. At this speed, the time difference between one gamma-ray hitting a more closely placed detector and that hitting one tens of centimetres further way is minute and not fully resolvable electronically. In most machines, an electronic time window can be set such that events recorded within a nanosecond time frame are regarded as occurring simultaneously. Recording such simultaneous events is the primary function of the tomograph. Any simultaneously recorded signal recorded from the two detectors indicates the occurrence of a positron annihilation. Singly detected events can arise from extraneous radiation, from positron annihilations occurring outside the field of view subtended by the two detectors, or because one or other of the two gamma rays has been stopped, or deflected from its path at 180° to the other.

Annihilation coincidence detection therefore provides an electronically determined precise field of view with uniform sensitivity. This is because wherever the disintegration takes place between the two detectors, for the event to be recorded the gamma rays must in sum have travelled the full interdetector distance. A single photon-emitting tracer, e.g. ^{99}Tc, ^{123}I or ^{133}Xe, cannot be quantified because the detectors view an ill-defined field with a sensitivity that decreases logarithmically from the detector face. The final problem is the question of deflection or stopping (attenuation) of the gamma rays by tissue, when the disintegration is occurring in the human body. With PET the correction for such attentuation can be directly measured for each plane of tissue studied and therefore accurately corrected. This involves making positron transmission measurements with an external source of a positron emitter prior to introduction of the relevant tracer into the body. Inaccuracies are introduced if this method of attenuation correction is not used. It is not possible with SPECT, a further major limitation of this considerably cheaper technique for physiological imaging in man.

Aspects of tomograph design which must be considered in evaluating the realization of the potential for quantification with PET include (a) detector efficiency and size; (b) the configuration of the detectors and the method used for maximizing sampling efficiency; (c) the speed of the electronic apparatus, its capacity to deal with the large count rates encountered in some studies, as well as means for distinguishing true from random coincidence counts.

A newer design variation is known as time-of-flight (TOF). This method attempts to use time discrimination of the arrival of the paired gamma rays at their respective detectors to place the disintegration in the space between them. This improves sensitivity but has a number of trade-off disadvantages. It is not clear at present that this represents a major breakthrough in instrumental design.

Once recorded, the data are computer processed by recognized and well-established tomographic reconstruction techniques which result in tomographic distributions of isotope concentrations with resolution characteristics dependent on the design of the individual tomograph used. Cameras are available with practical resolutions ranging from 17 × 17 × 17 mm³ to 5 × 5 × 7 mm³ resolution, which probably represents close to the maximal achievable practical resolution. Resolution is important only because the accuracy of an isotope concentration reading from a given structure depends on the size and homogeneity of the structure. To obtain a true reading, the structure should have a size twice the resolution element. Smaller structures will have their tracer concentration underestimated by a predictable amount, provided the size and shape of the structure is known. This means that the better the resolution, the more accurate will be the regional information.

TRACERS

The longest-lived gamma-emitting forms of oxygen, carbon, and nitrogen are all positron emitters. This means that naturally occurring molecules are potentially traceable with no alteration of molecular and therefore biological properties—a considerable advantage. However, despite being the longest-lived isotopes of these natural building blocks, they are nevertheless all very short-lived, e.g. the half-life of oxygen-15 (^{15}O) is 123 s, carbon-11 (^{11}C) 20.1 min, and nitrogen-13 (^{13}N) 10 min. In addition to these elements, rubidium-81 and -82 (^{81}Rb, ^{82}Rb) are biologically potassium analogues, one with a longer and the other a very short half-life. Fluorine-18 (^{18}F) has a half-life of 110 min and behaves when introduced into smaller molecules like the proton and so tends to be used as a hydrogen substitute. It has a comparatively longer half-life which makes it potentially transportable from a distant site of production to the PET facility. Indeed some PET centres transport ^{18}F-labelled compounds hundreds of miles by aircraft if they do not have a means of producing positron emitters themselves. A means of producing these isotopes at the site of usage is essential to have the capability of producing a wide range of tracers and labelled ligands. A modern cyclotron is therefore necessary, and this is the single most important disadvantage of investigating disease with PET. The capital and running costs are large and this means that such facilities are likely to remain in the research rather than routine clinical sphere for a considerable time to come.

PHYSIOLOGICAL MODELLING

The use of a labelled ligand to measure a physiological process depends on an understanding of the fate of the injected molecule and a description of the whole process in mathematical terms. I will use two examples to illustrate this concept: the steady-state oxygen inhalation method used to measure CBF, $CMRO_2$, and OER and the deoxyglucose method used to measure CMRGlc.

Oxygen metabolism

This method capitalizes on the short half-life of the ^{15}O label (123 s) and the biological properties of water in the human brain to measure CBF (the supply of oxygen to the brain), OER (the cerebral fractional extraction of oxygen from the perfusing arterial blood for the purposes of aerobic glucose metabolism), and $CMRO_2$ (the rate of utilization of oxygen by the brain). The conceptual model is simple. Inhalation of trace quantities of ^{15}O-labelled carbon dioxide gas ($C^{15}O_2$) is used to label water in the pulmonary capillary circulation *in vivo*. This is a rapid complete process which is facilitated by pulmonary capillary carbonic anhydrase and the principle of mass action:

$$C^{15}O_2 + H_2O \leftrightharpoons H_2C^{15}O_3 \leftrightharpoons H_2^{15}O + CO_2$$

The tracer thus becomes $H_2^{15}O$ in the circulation. This is swept into the left heart and distributed to the arterial circulation in general, as a functon of blood flow. Thus approximately 20 per cent arrives in the carotid and vertebral arteries and is then distributed throughout the cerebral capillary circulation. In the capillaries, the water diffuses rapidly into the tissues being completely extracted, whence it diffuses back into the venous capillary circulation and is swept away again to the heart. The water partitions equally between tissue and blood. If inhalation of $C^{15}O_2$ is continuous, the supply of $H_2^{15}O$ to the tissues is likewise. Because the half-life of the ^{15}O label is of the order of the transit time of H_2O through the cerebral circulation, label is rapidly decaying as well as being washed out of tissue where it has been deposited by the arterial blood. A steady state is achieved within three half-lives when the cerebral tissue $H_2^{15}O$ concentration becomes constant. This constant level represents a balance between delivery of tracer and loss by radioactive decay and flow through the tissue. Thus, if in the steady state the arterial concentration (delivery) and tissue concentration can be measured, CBF can be calculated. It is evident that if the PET camera and well counter used for measuring blood radioactivity can be cross-calibrated, the simple mathematical relationship is solvable regionally for CBF.

The subject is then made to breath molecular oxygen labelled with ^{15}O ($^{15}O_2$). In this instance the lung is used as an *in vivo* synthesizer of traces of ^{15}O-labelled oxyhaemoglobin ($Hb^{15}O_4$) This moiety is again distributed through the arterial tree, but in this instance only a certain proportion of the oxygen (^{15}O) is released and taken up by the tissues for oxidative metabolism. Normally this is about 30–40 per cent, the remaining 60 per cent or so passing through the capillary into the venous system unused. The oxygen in the tissues acts as an electron acceptor at the end of the cytochrome chain with the resulting formation of water, i.e. $H_2^{15}O$. In this case the tissue radioactivity is due to $H_2^{15}O$ produced metabolically in the tissue, rather than delivered from the circulation. The PET tissue ^{15}O activity measurement during continuous inhalation is however not purely due to metabolically produced water, but is contaminated by $Hb^{15}O_4$ which passes unextracted through the vasular space, and also $H_2^{15}O$ produced metabolically in all the body tissues which gets washed out into the venous circulation, whence it recirculates behaving like the circulating $H_2^{15}O$ produced by $C^{15}O_2$ inhalation and distributing according to the CBF. These two contaminating signals can be extracted to give the pure tissue metabolically generated $H_2^{15}O$ component which then allows simple calculation of OER. The blood volume (CBV) component can be extracted and corrected by measuring the CBV with a non-diffusing tracer such as ^{15}O- or ^{11}C-labelled carbon monoxide ($C^{15}O$ or ^{11}CO) inhaled in trace quantities. The information from the prior $C^{15}O_2$ inhalation with appropriate plasma and whole blood ^{15}O activity measurements can be used to correct for the recirculating $H_2^{15}O$ component. The product of CBF, OER, and the stable arterial oxygen content is the $CMRO_2$ which can therefore also be derived.

Thus, one label (^{15}O) and essentially one tracer ($H_2^{15}O$), though generated in two ways, are used to measure three variables, CBF, OER, and $CMRO_2$. The addition of a CO measurement allows CBV to be quantified and the measurement of OER and $CMRO_2$ to be made more accurate.

The advantages of this method are its conceptual, practical, and mathematical simplicity, its applicability to PET cameras unable to sample data quickly or with great efficiency and its reproducibility. A different approach to the same measurements with fast efficient cameras is to derive time-related data on the passage of a bolus of $C^{15}O_2$ and $^{15}O_2$ through the brain. If this can be done accurately, which presents technical problems, the need for a steady-state equilibrium method recedes, and quicker measurements are possible. The mathematical description of such a bolus technique is more complicated but still relatively simple and the method requires blood and tissue activity measurements with an acurate temporal resolution.

Glucose metabolism

A second and entirely different tracer strategy has been employed for measuring glucose consumption in the brain. This is an extention of a technique originally described for use with autoradiographic measurements of radioactivity in tissue slices in experimental animals. The use of PET to make the activity measurements has led for this reason to the use of the term *in vivo* autoradiography.

The problem with measuring a biochemical process *in vivo* with a radioactive tracer is how to ensure that the measured activity is all coming from the metabolite of interest. Glucose when taken up from the blood enters the glycolytic pathway at hexokinase whence it can pass to the Krebs cycle, be stored as glycogen, be used in synthesis of a number of intermediate metabolites, or be metabolized to lactate. The processes are fast and the products of such metabolism are labile. In the brain there is minimal, if any, capacity for glycogen production or intermediate metabolism and the vast majority enters the Krebs cycle for the production of ATP. The product of this pathway is CO_2 which is rapidly cleared from the tissue. This is the principal reason why ^{11}C-labelled glucose is an extremely difficult if not impossible tracer to use. The ^{11}C label disappears during the measurement and account of it cannot readily be made.

An alternative is to use a glucose *analogue* to study glycolytic flux. This should be transported across the blood–brain barrier (BBB) by the same mechanism as glucose and then metabolized by glycolysis but with a product that is trapped. Deoxyglucose is such an analogue. It uses the same BBB carrier mechanism as glucose and acts as a substrate for hexokinase. The product of this reaction is deoxyglucose 6-phosphate which is then trapped in the cerebral tissues because it cannot be metabolized further by the next enzyme in the glycolytic pathway. The brain is singular in that it contains no significant functional dephosphorylase either, so that the product of the hexokinase reaction cannot re-enter the precursor pool. The accumulation of deoxyglucose thus faithfully reflects the flux through hexokinase. If the handling of the analogue can be related to that of glucose in this chain of events, then the measure of deoxyglucose consumption should be directly translatable into that of glucose consumption, i.e. CMRGlc. This relationship is measurable and found to be constant under a wide variety of conditions—it is termed the lumped constant because it incorporates terms relating the different rates of transport and phosphorylation of the analogue and glucose. This relationship may break down in certain pathological states which seriously disrupt the structural integrity of the tissue. The CMRGlc is a measure of glycolytic flux which does not distinguish aerobic metabolism from that to lactate.

Translated into practice, the method involves measurement of blood–time activity curves, glucose concentration, and tissue concentration, and tissue activity (with PET) at steady state. The technique is practical and simple and because the ^{18}F label can be used to mark the deoxyglucose it has been widely used, as it is transportable to PET units without cyclotron facilities.

Both CMRGlc and CMRO$_2$ have been extensively used to study cerebral function because of the clear demonstration in animal work of a close and linear relationship between neuronal function and local metabolic activity. The combination of metabolic and blood flow markers has been especially useful in the study of cerebral disease. In particular the haemodynamic and energy balance relationships in stroke, cerebrovascular disease, and cerebral tumours have been explored. The concurrent measurement of CMRO$_2$ and CMRGlc can be used to dissect out the proportions of oxidative and non-oxidative metabolism of glucose by calculation of the stoichiometric relationship between the two.

From this brief description of the concepts involved in two well-established and verified tracer techniques applied to man by the use of PET measurement, it is clear that the study of biochemical and physiological processes *in vivo* is a reality. The development of methods is not easy. It involves a multitude of steps requiring a wide variety of expertise—biochemists to indicate tracers of interest, radiochemists to synthesize labelled tracers, physiologists to describe the behaviour of the tracers in terms of blood–brain barrier passage, metabolic fate, distribution, and compartmentalization. These processes must then be mathematically described and practically possible measurements defined, sufficient to allow solution of the mathematical model for the variable under study.

PSYCHIATRIC APPLICATIONS

The strategies and options at present available for the study of psychiatric disease are limited. With haemodynamics and energy metabolism, one is driven to observations of secondary phenomena of an indirect nature. Systematic studies of normal energy metabolism and blood flow as well as focal changes in response to specific stimuli have been well documented. Their attenuation in pathological states such as dementias, schizophrenias, or depressions have not been studied. Of the studies of energy metabolism in schizophrenia, many have been comparatively inconclusive. No major site of focal pathology has been demonstratd though there are indications of altered relationships between different regions and right/left hemispheric asymmetries (see Chapters 3, 4, and 6.)

The response of the brain to medication has been little studied. Energy metabolism and blood flow can be monitored with considerable precision in pre- and post-medication states. A number of preliminary reports indicating alteration of physiological parameters before and after therapeutic intervention have been communicated in cerebrovascular diseases, the dementias (see Chapter 7), and parkinsonism.

A more direct approach might be investigation of neurotransmitter systems. In the last year or so radiochemists have provided ^{18}F- and ^{11}C-labelled L -dopa and spiperone, a dopamine receptor antagonist. Scans in humans have shown specific uptake of the tracer in dopamine-receptor-rich regions such as the striatum, and little or no uptake into those areas relatively free of such receptors, e.g. the cerebellum. The initial distribution of tracer is non-specific and largely blood-flow-determined but with the passage of time, the tracer is washed out of areas of non-specific binding whilst concentrating in areas of specific uptake. L -dopa and spiperone are well suited for such studies as both bind with avidity and with a long time course.

The opiate system is now also coming under study with reports of specific binding of ^{11}C-labelled buprenorphine to thalamic and frontal areas. Other opiate ligands are being labelled and their PET-recorded distribtions awaited eagerly. The modelling required to make sense of these PET-recorded distributions is complicated, and still in early developmental phases. The hope is that receptor densities and binding characteristis may be quantifiable at some future date. This activity is of great interest to those who think that psychiatric disorders may have a basis in specific neurotransmitter system dysfunction, and clinical studies are in progress.

The pharmacokinetic study of psychoactive drug metabolism, distribution, and binding is also a feasible endeavour. It again depends on labelling the ligands and an awareness of metabolic pathways. The measurement of the time course of ligand concentrations in different brain regions might give clues to the sites of action or indirectly indicate receptor densities for the various types of psychoactive agent. A number of possible lines of experimentation include measuring distributions before and after various concentrations of cold ligand, and binding displacement studies. The distribution of many drugs in the human brain *in vivo* are quite unknown and this technique provides a potential means for investigating such problems.

Much optimism has been generated in those who feel that the only reason organic bases for the various psychiatric syndromes have not been elucidated has been the lack of a suitable investigative tool. It remains to be seen whether syndromes such as schizophrenia can indeed be described in terms of specific neurotransmitter system dysfunction. It is probable that PET is the investigative technique of choice for research of such hypotheses in man.

CONCLUSIONS

PET is a technique for measuring regional radiotracer distributions in the brain *in vivo*. It has imaging capabilities because the method of data collection and analysis involves classical tomographic reconstruction techniques. Quantitative measurement of a limited number of physiological and biochemical variables is already possible. The study of neurotransmitter systems appears to be possible from preliminary distribution data in the dopaminergic and opiate systems.

The clinical application of PET has had its greatest impact thus far on neurological diseases such as cerebrovascular disease, epilepsy (see Chapter 6), aging and dementia (see Chapter 7), and cerebral tumours, where new physiological observations of basic clinical and therapeutic importance have been made. Some of these observations are being translated into clinical practice, notably in the management of extracranial occlusive vascular disease and the reassessment of the role of tumour ischaemia in resistance to radiotherapy. The application of PET to the study of psychiatric disease is in its infancy. Studies are under way and the next few years should see the answers to a number of current hypotheses concerning their pathogenesis and pharmacotherapy. Of particular interest in this line is a recent report by Reiman and co-workers of a non-dominant parahippocampal focal abnormality which seems to correlate with a syndrome of lactate-induced panic attacks. If focal dysfunction like this is indeed confirmed and indicates a pathogenic phenomenon, then considerable weight will accrue to the biological hypotheses of the aetiology of psychiatric disease.

SUGGESTED READING

A highly selected introductory reading list is provided which should complement the reference lists of the other chapters in this monograph dealing with PET studies in human disease.

Ell, P. J. and Holman, B. L. (eds) (1982). *Computed emission tomography*. Oxford University Press, Oxford, pp. 1–546.
Frackowiak, R. S. J. and Wise, R. J. S. (1983). Positron tomography in ischaemic cerebrovascular disease. *Neurol. Clin.* **1(1)**, 183–201.
—— Lenzi, G. L., Jones, T., and Heather, J. D. (1980). Quantitative measurement of regional cerebral blood flow and oxygen metabolism in man using ^{15}O and positron

emission tomography: theory, procedure and normal values. *J. Comput. Assist. Tomogr.* **14**, 727–36.

—— Pozzilli, C., Legg, N. J., DuBoulay, G. H., Marshall, J., Lenzi, G. L., and Jones, T. (1981). Regional cerebral oxygen supply and utilisation in dementia: a clinical and physiological study with oxygen-15 and positron tomography. *Brain* **104**, 753–78.

Gibbs, J. M., Wise, R. J. S., Leenders, K. L., and Jones, T. (1984). Evaluation of cerebral perfusion reserve in patients with carotid artery occlusion. *Lancet* **i**, 310–14.

Heiss, W. D. and Phelps, M. E. (eds) (1983). *Positron emission tomography of the brain.* Springe Verlag, New York.

Leenders, K. L., Herold, S., Brooks, D. J., Palmer, A. J., Turton, D., Firnau, G., Garnett, E. S., Nahmias, C., and Veall, N. (1984). Presynaptic and post-synaptic dopaminergic system in human brain, *Lancet* **ii**, 110–11.

Magistretti, P. L. (ed.) (1983). *Functional radionuclide imaging of the brain.* Raven Press, New York, pp. 253–368.

Mazziotta, J. C., Phelps, M. E., Carson, R. E., and Kuhl, D. E. (1982). Tomographic mapping of human cerebral metabolism. Sensory deprivation. *Ann. Neurol.* **12**, 435–44.

—— —— —— and —— (1982). Tomographic mapping of human cerebral metabolism: auditory stimulation. *Neurology* **12**, 435–44.

—— —— Miller, J., and Kuhl, D. E. (1981). Tomographic mapping of human cerebral metabolism: Normal unstimulated state. *Neurology* **31**, 503–16.

Phelps, M. E. (1977). Emission computed tomography. *Semin. Nucl. Med.* **7**, 337–65.

—— Mazziotta, J. C., and Huang, S. C. (1982). Study of cerebral function with positron computed tomography. *J. Cereb. Blood Flow Metab.* **2**, 113–62.

—— Huang, S. C., Hoffman, E. J., Selin, E. J., Sokoloff, L., and Kuhl, D. E. (1979). Tomographic measurement of local cerebral glucose metabolic rate in humans with (F-18) 2-fluoro-2-deoxy-D glucose: Validation of method. *Ann. Neurol.* **6**, 371–88.

—— Mazziotta, J. C., Kuhl, D. E., Nuwer, M., Packwood, J., Metter, J., and Engel, J., Jr. (1981). Tomographic mapping of human cerebral metabolism: Visual stimulation and deprivation. *Neurology* **31**, 517–29.

Reiman, E. M., Raichle, M. E., Butler, F. K., Herscovitch, P., and Robins, E. (1984). A local brain abnormality in panic disorder, a severe form of anxiety. *Nature, Lond.* **310**, 683–5.

Sheppard, G., Gruzelier, J., Manchada, R., Hirsch, S. R., Wise, R., Frackowiak, R. S. J., and Jones, T. (1983). ^{15}O positron emission tomography scanning in predominantly never-treated acute schizophrenic patients. *Lancet* **ii**, 1448–52.

Sokoloff, L. (1981). Localisation of functional activity in the cerebral nervous system by measurement of glucose utilisation with radioactive deoxyglucose. *J. Cereb. Blood Flow Metab.* **1**, 7–36.

Ter-Pogassian, M. M. (1981). Special characteristics and potential for dynamic function studies with PET. *Semin. Nucl. Med.* **11** 13–23.

Wagner, H. N., Burns, D. H., Dannals, R. F., Wong, D. F., Langstrom, B., Duelfero, T., Frost, J. J., Ravert, H. T., Kings, J. M., Rosenbloom, S. B., Lukas, S. E., Kramer, A. V., and Kuhar, M. J. (1984). Imaging dopamine receptors in the brain by positron tomography. *Science* **221**, 1264–6.

3

Positron emission tomographic studies in schizophrenia: a review

MICHAEL R. SMITH AND JONATHAN D. BRODIE

INTRODUCTION

The application of a complex technology such as positron emission tomography (PET) to the study of brain function in psychopathological states poses a series of problems and challenges which may be loosely termed 'methodological'. Research structure and interpretation in biological psychiatry has been limited by problems associated with diagnoses based on behavioural phenomenology, small subject populations, psychotropic drug effects, differing experimental designs, and state vs trait distinctions. A host of factors peculiar to PET of which the general scientific community may not be aware include: (1) metabolic and modelling assumptions, (2) the distortions introduced by technical problems associated with the inherent resolution of the scanner in relation to the size of the anatomical region of interest (ROI), (3) the methods of data collection and the strategies of image analysis, and (4) the metabolic consequences of the experimental conditions (such as sensory deprivation). In addition, the determination of the accuracy, precision and reproducibility of the reconstructed data has yet to be satisfactorily determined in experimental populations subjected to various manoeuvres and important details. These include reproducible head positioning, and the inherent variance in skull and cerebral anatomy, which can cause marked changes in the position of a given anatomical structure in the brain of different subjects. Although it is not possible to explore all of these issues in a short article, we shall illustrate some of them as they apply to the study of psychiatric disorders in the context of the application of PET in the study of the schizophrenic syndrome. This chapter does not purport to be a comprehensive review of all studies performed to date, many of which are in the publication process, but is meant to be a critical review.

The application of PET to the study of schizophrenia had its origins in the findings of Ingvar and Franzen (1974) who used the classical xenon blood flow technique to compare the regional cortical blood flow of a small population of chronic schizophrenic subjects at rest without sensory deprivation to a group of chronic alcoholics who served as a control group. They found that flow in the frontal cortex of schizophrenics was diminished in comparison with the controls, giving rise to the term 'hypofrontality'. The PET studies we shall address use either labelled oxygen or glucose and its analogues as markers of neuronal energy metabolism under the metabolic assumptions that there is a direct coupling of blood flow and energy metabolism, and that all of these markers are measuring the same process and can be correlated by making appropriate kinetic corrections. These metabolic assumptions appear well founded (DiChiro *et al.* 1984) although the use of glucose analogues as markers of glucose utilization has been questioned (Sacks *et al.* 1983).

The general premise of PET studies with schizophrenics is that subjects with this illness will exhibit a pattern of regional energy metabolism which can distinguish them from 'normal' subjects. This expectation rests on the original flow studies of Kety and Schmidt (1948), the flow experiment of Lassen and Ingvar (1974), and the initial PET study of Farkas *et al.* (1980) on a single subject. Each of these studies were performed with unstimulated (i.e. 'resting') conditions, although clearly the experimental conditions were quite different in each of the laboratories. Subsequent PET studies used a cross-sectional design in which small groups of subjects who met defined diagnostic criteria were examined in a defined state (resting or stimulated), and metabolic scans of patients were compared with scans from normal subjects obtained under similar conditions (Widen *et al.* 1981; Buchsbaum *et al.* 1982; Sheppard *et al.* 1983; Farkas *et al.* 1984; Clark *et al.* 1984). Other studies modified the approach by using an intervention (either treatment or stimulation) and comparing two states within the same patient and with a normal population under similar conditions, if appropriate (Widen *et al.* 1983; Brodie *et al.* 1984; Wolkin *et al.* 1985). These studies are summarized in Table 3.1.

Although these studies represent a logical starting point, they underscore the difficulty in investigating this important syndrome since the patient population has been defined by criteria that allow for a great diversity of presentation. This heterogeneity may yet be addressed when the study groups become sufficiently large, but of the many dimensions which may contribute to the presentation only the acute/chronic dimension appears reasonably addressed. At the present time the relative contributions of positive and negative symptoms, duration of illness, premorbid adjustment, effects of medication and attentional and cognitive deficits have not been systematically approached, either within or among the various groups, although clinical experience would suggest that these factors would be significant.

On balance, the studies summarized in Table 3.1 would suggest that chronic schizophrenia is associated with a decrease in metabolism in the frontal lobes when compared with the rest of the brain, while acute schizophrenics and normal controls do not appear to show this relationship. This conclusion must be qualified by a number of considerations. Only one of the studies (Wolkin *et al.* 1985) analysed the data on an absolute metabolic activity basis, as well as a ratio or other correlational method, and studied the same patients before and after medication. Even then, this study did not address the effect of chronic medication on frontal lobe metabolism which is of crucial importance in determining whether frontal lobe metabolic activity changes are a consequence of the illness or its treatment.

RESEARCH DESIGNS

All of the studies listed in Table 3.1 make use of a cross-sectional design strategy in which an experimental group meeting a research criteria for schizophrenia is compared, on a variable relating to the cerebral uptake of a radiopharmaceutical, to a control group free of the disease. The two groups are then compared for 'statistically significant' differences.

The majority of the studies also include a description of how a particular variable related to cerebral metabolism is distributed among the subjects within the schizophrenic or normal groups. In two of the studies (Widen *et al.* 1983; Brodie *et al.* 1984), an uncontrolled longitudinal structure is employed in an attempt to determine how one variable (again a measure relating to cerebral metabolism) depends on a second (in both cases neuroleptic drug treatment).

Despite the pitfalls inherent in comparing experiments which differ greatly in execution and methods, some authors have sought to compare data obtained from the acute schizophrenic populations investigated (Widen *et al.* 1983; Sheppard *et al.* 1983) with results from the studies of more chronic schizophrenic groups (Widen *et al.* 1981; Brodie *et al.* 1984). When taken together in this fashion, the combined experiments form a longitudinal study in which the prevalence of a variable relating to cerebral metabolism is compared to the duration of the schizophrenic illness.

All of the studies reviewed share in non-random assignment of the independent variable under study (e.g. diagnosis, duration of illness). This is not to say that the random assignment of experimental conditions, such as psychiatric diagnosis, is practical, possible or desirable (Feinstein 1977). However, it should suggest caution in the interpretation of results, the 'significance' of which are generated by statistical methods (e.g. Students's t test, ANOVA) which assume a random distribution of error about the mean (Fisher 1966). The classical experimental model, which employs the random assignment of experimental conditions, restricts systematic bias or error and reduces the likelihood that statistical assumptions will be violated. The potential for Type I error (false rejection of the null hypothesis) is thereby reduced. Since the data generated by the early studies applying PET to the study of potential derangements of cerebral metabolism in schizophrenia have been viewed as 'hypothesis generating', it would clearly be advantageous to restrict the possibility of Type I errors which would in turn generate false hypotheses. Therefore, a cautious common sense approach to the statistical evaluation of metabolic data generated by the designs described above and employed by the cerebral metabolic studies of schizophrenia to date is preferable to the use of mathematically arcane 'tests of statistical significance' which do little to further the scientific or clinical understanding of the metabolic concomitants of psychiatric illness.

TABLE 3.1.

Study	Subjects and Methods	Findings	Conclusions
Widen et al. (1981)	Schizophrenics ($n = 8$); controls ($n = 2$); tracer = [^{11}C] glucose	Decreased frontal lobe glucose utilization in schizophrenic patients when expressed as a ratio between metabolic rate of frontal and temporal lobe regions of interest.	Abnormal distribution of cerebral metabolic activity in schizophrenia ('hypofrontality') supported.
Buchsbaum et al. (1982)	Schizophrenics ($n = 8$); controls ($n = 6$); tracer = [^{18}F]fluorodeoxyglucose; uptake conditions = eyes closed and ears plugged.	Decreased cortical glucose utilization in superior frontal lobes of schizophrenic patients; decreased left central grey matter uptake in schizophrenics.	Frontal cortex in schizophrenia has relatively low functional activity; basal ganglia dysfunction demonstrated in schizophrenic patients.
Widen et al. (1983)	Schizophrenics ($n = 6$) characterized by short duration of illness examined before and after treatment with neuroleptic drugs; controls ($n = 2$); tracer = [^{11}C] glucose	No significant differences in glucose utilization found between schizophrenic and control groups: left greater than right basal ganglia uptake of glucose in untreated schizophrenics which was abolished by neuroleptic treatment: decreased left frontal lobe glucose utilization results from treatment.	Chronicity of schizophrenic illness implicated as 'cause' of hypofrontal metabolic activity; neuroleptic drug treatment decreases asymmetry of basal ganglia uptake of glucose.
Sheppard et al. (1983)	Schizophrenics ($n = 12$); controls ($n = 12$) characterized by short duration of illness and minimal or no treatment with neuroleptic medication; tracers = ^{15}O$_2$ and C^{15}O$_2$; uptake conditions with eyes closed.	Schizophrenic group did not differ significantly from controls on indices of hypofrontal metabolism: as a group schizophrenics exhibited less left–right cerebral asymmetry.	'Hypofrontality hypothesis' not supported in a schizophrenic group lacking chronicity of illness and neuroleptic drug exposure: abnormality of cerebral laterality in schizophrenic group is a cause or effect of the illness.

Farkas et al. (1984)	Schizophrenics ($n = 13$); controls ($n = 11$); tracer = [^{18}F]fluorodeoxyglucose; uptake conditions = eyes closed.	Decreased frontal lobe metabolic activity in schizophrenic patients: medicated schizophrenics do not differ significantly from non-medicated schizophrenics in cerebral uptake of glucose.	Hypofrontal pattern of glucose metabolism is associated with schizophrenic illness.
Brodie et al. (1984)	Chronic schizophrenics ($n = 6$) examined before and after treatment with neuroleptic drugs; controls ($n = 5$); tracer = [^{18}F]fluorodeoxyglucose; uptake conditions = eyes open, ears plugged.	Frontal lobe metabolism decreased in an asymmetric pattern (left > right) in schizophrenic patients; treatment does not affect asymmetric pattern of frontal lobe uptake or frontal lobe hypometabolism.	Relative left frontal hypometabolism may be a physiological derangement characteristic of chronic schizophrenia and is unaffected by exposure to neuroleptic drugs.
Clark et al. (1984)	Schizophrenics ($n = 7$) examined off neuroleptic drugs; controls ($n = 9$); tracer = [^{18}F]fluorodeoxyglucose; uptake conditions = eyes closed, ears plugged with somatosensory stimulation (electric shocks) to right forearm.	The number of significant correlations between local metabolic rates within the schizophrenic and control groups exceeded chance expectancy; the number of significant correlations of local metabolic rates differed significantly between schizophrenics and controls.	Patterns of metabolic coupling between brain areas exist and conform with current understanding of brain function.
Wolkin et al. (1985)	Chronic schizophrenics ($n = 10$) examined before and after somatic treatment; controls ($n = 8$); tracer [^{18}F]fluorodeoxyglucose; uptake conditions = eyes open, ears plugged.	Pretreatment schizophrenic patients compared to controls had markedly lower absolute values of glucose uptake in frontal and temporal regions and relatively increased basal ganglia uptake; posttreatment metabolic rates approached normal values in all brain regions except the frontal lobes.	Frontal lobes confirmed as a specific locus of aberrant cerebral functioning in chronic schizophrenia: decreased metabolic activity in the temporal lobe area may be associated with chronic schizophrenia: persistent metabolic changes differentiate chronic schizophrenics from normals regardless of treatment effects.

SUBJECT SELECTION AND DIAGNOSIS

The problems in selection and diagnosis of subjects for biological psychiatry research devolve from issues pertaining to the reliability with which a particular diagnosis can be applied and the validity of the diagnostic criteria with respect to predictive power on factors such as genetic transmission, response to treatment, and long-term outcome. Modern psychiatric diagnostic criteria were developed primarily in response to the pragmatic concerns of research workers over the low reliability of diagnostic systems which did not contain explicit inclusion and exclusion criteria. Psychiatric diagnostic systems such as the research diagnostic criteria (RDC) of (Spitzer *et al.* (1978*a*)) have improved the reliability with which a particular diagnosis can be applied (Spitzer *et al.* 1978*b*). However, these same criteria have been criticized by some (Overall and Hollister 1979; Berner *et al.* 1983) who contend the validity of research diagnostic criteria is low in terms of their likelihood of selecting patients who conform with prevailing or classical clinical concepts of psychiatric illness, and that the use of a single diagnostic system for psychiatric research should be rejected. Therefore, in assembling groups of psychiatric patients for biological study, investigators must consider in the selection of a diagnostic system not only the reliability with which the conclusions reached from the study of their own groups can be extrapolated to the results obtained by other investigators, but also the degree to which the members of their own experimental group are representative of the patient population under study as a whole.

The studies reviewed in Table 3.1. are quite consistent in their diagnostic approach, all using either the RDC of Spitzer (Widen *et al.* 1981, 1983; Sheppard *et al.* 1983; Farkas *et al.* 1984; Brodie *et al.* 1984), the DSM III (American Psychiatric Association, 1980) (Clark *et al.* 1984; Wolkin *et al.* 1985) or both (Buchsbaum *et al.* 1982) as inclusion criteria for schizophrenic subjects. Both the RDC of Spitzer and the DSM III criteria for the schizophrenia derive from the St Louis RDC of Feighner *et al.* (1982) and are therefore quite similar conceptually. In both, symptomatological inclusion criteria consist of reported symptoms which correspond mainly to the first rank symptoms of Schneider (1959) and observed symptoms which stress the presence or absence of disordered thinking. The two systems differ primarily in their exclusion criteria for duration of illness and presence of affective disorder. DSM III requires 6 months of continuous symptomatology for the diagnosis of schizophrenia compared to 2 weeks for the RDC. A RDC diagnosis of schizophrenia cannot be made if cross-sectional criteria for major affective illness are met, while the DSM III permits a diagnosis of schizophrenia in this situation if the major affective symptoms developed after the onset of psychosis. Hence, in comparing results from studies using the two different diagnostic systems, one could expect the schizophrenic groups to differ substantially in terms of chronicity of illness and presence or absence of affective symptomatology. Since these factors (chronic course, absence of affective symptoms) have been associated clinically with poor prognosis and resistance to conventional treatment (process schizophrenia), the expected differences in experimental populations diagnosed under the two systems assumes more than technical importance.

It is interesting to note that, in the single study which presented detailed diagnostic information (Buchsbaum *et al.* 1982), of the eight 'schizophrenic' patients studied, three did not meet RDC and two did not meet DSM III criteria for schizophrenia—the exceptions in all cases receiving a diagnosis of schizoaffective disorder. Since the RDC and DSM III presumably restrict the diagnosis of schizophrenia in the presence of affective symptomatology in an attempt to reduce overlap between the two diagnostic groups, the inclusion of patients diagnosed as schizoaffective in a group of 'schizophrenics' assembled for the purpose of delineating metabolic concomitants of the illness merits some concern. This diagnostic issue, not trivial when one considers the proportion of schizoaffective subjects included in the study, has made the results of the study difficult to interpret and compare.

In summary, agreement on the use of a single diagnostic system by all investigators engaged in research work on small samples of patients should be encouraged. If it is felt that the use of a single diagnostic system is too restrictive for the purposes of the research, the experimental group meeting criteria for the single system adopted should be treated separately at some point in the data analysis to allow for comparisons between experimental results.

EXPERIMENTAL CONDITIONS

It is generally considered crucial in any study of brain function to be able to control experimental conditions. Control of intrasubject variation in endogenous cerebral activity is complicated by the long temporal base of PET experiments relative to the actual physiological duration of neural events estimated to be in the millisecond time range. The temporal resolution for quantitative PET imaging is limited by the number of radioactive events required for accurate reconstruction of the metabolic image, which in turn depends on the acceptable radiation dose for human subjects undergoing a non-therapeutic procedure, and the tracer and kinetic model employed.

In their present state, each of the markers of energy consumption has unique problems when used with PET. Because the fidelity of the image is based in part on the counting statistics, and this is a scalar function, in general it takes at least several minutes to achieve acceptable precision without using tracer levels causing radiation danger. The use of labelled glucose has the drawback that due to its rapid metabolism and distribution by glycolysis and metabolism in the tricarboxylic acid cycle, appropriate modelling for quantitative measurements has not yet been achieved for the time frame necessitated by instruments presently in use. On the other hand it has the advantage of being a direct tracer of energy consumption since it accounts for greater than 90 per cent of the metabolizable substrate for neuronal energy requirements (Sokoloff 1981). Oxygen, or oxygen-labelled water, have been used quite effectively in a quantitative fashion (Frackowiak *et al.* 1980), but because of the 2 min half-life and rapid distribution it cannot be used with high resolution and give quantitative neuroanatomical fidelity for smaller brain regions.

2-[^{18}F]Fluorodeoxyglucose (FDG) and 2-[^{11}C]deoxyglucose (CDG) have the advantage of unambiguous localization because of the metabolic trap and a refined mathematical model (Huang *et al.* 1980) but the major disadvantage of requiring a long uptake period (*ca.* 40 min) before the requirements of the model are met. Direct comparison of studies using different tracers, and necessarily different physical and temporal constraints, must be made with caution. Because of the long temporal resolution of PET measurements relative to the duration of the cerebral neuronal processes to which they relate, the actual usefulness of decreasing temporal resolution by even a factor of ten in terms of minutes is questionable unless stimulation studies of the experimental subject are planned. In which case, a reduction in non-task-related cerebral activity, such as distraction by extraneous stimuli, poor motivation, and habituation, may be desirable. In such a case a tracer strategy with superior temporal resolution would be advantageous.

Since endogenous cerebral activity is, on a subjective basis, obviously extremely variable between individuals and between such groups as schizophrenic patients and normal controls, the resting state has been criticized by many as being an unsuitable reference state because of the lack of control over the subject's mental activity. Curiously, there has been no report as yet of the long-term stability of PET measures under these or any other conditions. However, a short-term (same day) test/retest strategy using CDG in a normal population (Russell *et al.* unpublished work) shows a surprisingly good stability with an eyes open, ears plugged resting state (variance = 5 per cent in most brain regions).

Hence, the stability of PET measures of cerebral activity in the light of such variables as the endogenous mental and emotional state of the experimental subject is unclear. Since it is unlikely that a design strategy can be implemented which would control for such subjective mental processes, the interpretations of findings of systematic variation in cerebral metabolism between experimental groups composed of psychiatrically ill patients and normal controls must be tempered by an appreciation of the lack of control over such variables—until it is shown how such variables affect quantitative PET measures.

Resting-state studies have been shown in normal subjects to be, within some limits, quite affected by variables over which experimental control can be exerted, such as sensory stimulation or deprivation (Mazziotta *et al.* 1983). It has been reported (Mazziotta and Phelps 1984) that marked reduction of both auditory and visual input leads to predominantly right-sided metabolic hypometabolism, while either plugging of the ears or blindfolding the subject does not cause this effect. Since hypothetical explanations for these findings centre around functional morphological or biochemical asymmetries, one or both of which could conceivably be altered in schizophrenia, these studies may not accurately reflect the responses of a schizophrenic population which may not only vary on morphological or biochemical variables, but also, particularly in a hallucinatory state, on the relative level of sensory deprivation achieved. Even so, a systematic attempt to resolve the question of resting state conditions on metabolic activity in schizophrenic patients has not been attempted nor has a uniform approach to the examination of subjects, which would make results from the various studies more easily comparable, been instituted. Some of the studies summarized in Table 3.1 were performed with subjects who had their eyes open and ears plugged (Brodie *et al.* 1984; Wolkin *et al.* 1985), some in the reverse condition (Farkas *et al.* 1984; Sheppard *et al.* 1983) and one (Buchsbaum *et al.* 1982) was carried out under conditions of sensory deprivation. These considerations make even the 'resting-state' comparisons problematic and may have a profound effect on results analysed for lateral asymmetry.

IMAGE AND DATA ANALYSIS

Because of the problems associated with the analysis of the images and raw data generated by a typical PET study, a multiplicity of approaches have evolved out of the attempt to reliably and objectively characterize aberrant cerebral functioning in groups of patients exhibiting symptoms of schizophrenia. Image analysis strategies can be classified according to their methods of anatomical localization and mathematical expression of the raw metabolic data. Anatomical loci may be defined by so-called 'objective' methods in which mathematical criteria are used to define cerebral regions of interest (ROI) for subsequent data analysis, or by more 'subjective' strategies in which ROIs are independently determined using the subject's CT scan as an anatomical reference. The raw metabolic data contained within a particular plane of section or ROI can then be expressed as an average absolute value, as a quotient relating regional uptake to a corresponding global or regional metabolic value or as a statistic such as covariance with another brain region.

Considering first the specifics of the anatomical localization schemes which have been adopted in the studies reviewed, all share a common point of departure which involves the identification of the anatomical plane of section represented by a particular metabolic image. Because of the anatomical variance of skull and intracerebral structures, subject movement and variations in positioning from one subject to another, reliance on a single criterion such as distance above the initial plane of section has not been used to identify the anatomical plane of section with two exceptions (Buchsbaum *et al.* 1982; Sheppard *et al.* 1983). Even if one ignores error generated by subject anatomical variation and positioning inaccuracies, a comparison of these two studies is further complicated by their use of different reference planes (canthomeatal and orbitomeatal) which, because of the fifteen degree angulation between them, would have profound effects on the anatomical structures included in a particular section which lies a significant distance from the centre of the anatomical plane of reference. Since the two studies report conflicting findings, one wonders how much the comparison would be influenced by a correction for the difference in anatomical structures studied in a given plane of section. In the remainder of the studies, identification of cerebral structures was accomplished by independent comparison to a CT scan in the same plane of section or by the use of standard referent PET images. In all of the studies the anatomical planes of section derived from the first step of the image analysis were further divided into discrete regions of interest. This was accomplished by transferring anatomical areas outlined on CT scan directly to the PET image (Widen *et al.* 1983), by visual comparison of the CT scan corresponding to the PET image (Farkas *et al.* 1984; Brodie *et al.* 1984), and arbitrarily by the use of computer-generated mathematically-derived mapping techniques (Buchsbaum *et al.* 1982; Sheppard *et al.* 1983) or subjective placement of the anatomical ROI directly on the metabolic image (Sheppard *et al.*; Clark *et al.* 1984). The number of ROIs into which a particular anatomical plane is divided varies between two (Farkas *et al.* 1984) and 34 (Sheppard *et al.* 1983). The size and contour of the selected ROIs are particularly important with the low-resolution first- and second-generation scanners with which the present studies were performed, since the relatively large partial volume effects lead to a blurring of the image and even a loss of quantification (Budinger *et al.* 1984). In summary, the reports in Table 3.1 reflect not only varying strategies and degrees of subjectivity in defining ROIs, but also an inconsistent approach to combining the geometry of the ROI with the technical limitations imposed by the scanners employed. This has the effect of making conclusions drawn from comparisons between the findings of different groups (e.g. hypofrontality as a concomitant of chronic but not acute schizophrenia) difficult.

Returning to an evaluation of the methods employed in the analysis of the raw metabolic data derived from the image analysis, we are again confronted by a somewhat bewildering variety of approaches. For example, the term 'hypofrontal' was originally used to describe the cerebral blood flow pattern in schizophrenics. This necessarily only reflects cortical activity because of the limitations of that technique. Some workers (Farkas *et al.* 1984; Brodie *et al.* 1984) have used the term to mean the relationship of frontal cortical activity to the activity of the brain in the plane of section, while others (Buchsbaum *et al.* 1982; Widen *et al.* 1983) have used the term in the original sense. Although there is merit in considering the entire plane of section, thus addressing cortical–subcortical relationships, some confusion has been introduced as a result of using the same term to describe different analyses.

The problem of using relative metabolic values to identify possible cerebral changes in schizophrenia is illustrated by comparing the results of Widen *et al.* (1983), who examined a small sample of six acute

TABLE 3.2. *Mean absolute regional* CMRGlc (glucose consumption) ±S.E.M. *by subject group schizophrenics* (*Wolkin* et al. *1985*).

ROI MV slice		Normal	Pretreatment	Posttreatment
Whole		32.9 ± 1.1	29.2 ± 0.8*	33.2 ± 1.7
L	hemislice	33.7 ± 1.1	29.4 ± 0.9**	33.4 ± 1.7
R	hemislice	32.1 ± 1.2	29.1 ± 0.8*	33.0 ± 1.7
L	frontal cortex	35.3 ± 1.7	28.4 ± 1.2***	31.1 ± 2.6
R	frontal cortex	33.7 ± 2.0	29.3 ± 1.4	32.0 ± 2.8
L	posterior	33.6 ± 1.1	29.7 ± 1.0*	34.0 ± 1.5
R	posterior	32.0 ± 1.1	29.3 ± 0.9	33.7 ± 1.4*
L	temporal cortex	34.6 ± 1.5	28.4 ± 1.1***	32.9 ± 1.8
R	temporal cortex	34.0 ± 1.1	29.1 ± 1.2**	34.2 ± 1.8*
L	caudate	34.1 ± 1.5	33.6 ± 1.8	36.9 ± 2.6
R	caudate	30.3 ± 1.7	30.4 ± 1.4	33.9 ± 2.1
L	lenticular	40.8 ± 1.2	38.0 ± 1.1	42.6 ± 2.3
R	lenticular	36.5 ± 1.6	36.6 ± 1.2	40.1 ± 2.3
L	occipital cortex	32.3 ± 1.8	29.0 ± 1.4	35.4 ± 1.9*
R	occipital cortex	33.0 ± 1.6	30.4 ± 1.6	37.0 ± 2.1

Medication-free schizophrenics had significantly lower (20%) absolute regional metabolic rates of glucose utilization than the normal group in the left frontal ($P < 0.005$) and the left ($P < 0.005$) and right ($P < 0.01$) temporal cortex in the mid-ventricular plane. There was an overall increase in glucose utilization after treatment. Hypofrontality is defined in spatial terms as the ratio of the CMR glucose in the frontal lobes to the rest of the brain in the plane of section, is observed in this group of patients both before and after treatment. With the exception of the frontal/posterior ratio, which further decreased after treatment, there was no gross change in the metabolic pattern.

    * $P < 0.05$
    ** $P < 0.01$
    *** $P < 0.005$

schizophrenics and two controls, and the study of Wolkin *et al.* (1985), who compared ten chronic schizophrenics and eight controls (see Table 3.2).

The frontal/temporal ratio analysis of Widen showed that unmedicated acute schizophrenics were indistinguishable from his small control group. The results of Wolkin, which in absolute terms showed a marked decrease in frontal ($P < 0.01$) and temporal lobe ($P < 0.005$) metabolism, would have shown a result similar to that found by Widen if presented as a ratio. Likewise, after medication, both studies showed diminished frontal/temporal ratios, but, as found in the Wolkin study, this was because the metabolic response to neuroleptic administration was greater in the temporal lobe than in the frontal lobe in absolute metabolic terms.

When one extends these considerations of image and data analysis to include differences in experimental conditions and subject populations, it is easier to appreciate why the findings of two groups can have results that appear to be similar, but in fact are quite different. The laboratories of New York University-Brookhaven National Laboratories (NYU-BNL) and the

National Institute of Health (NIH) both report hypofrontality in small groups of schizophrenics compared to normal. However, the NIH group found that this is significant in the superior frontal cortex while the NYU-BNL group found no significant difference in this region and did find that the middle and inferior frontal regions were hypometabolic. Because virtually every important aspect of the experiments were performed differently, these findings are not readily reconcilable.

FUTURE DIRECTIONS

With all of the caveats and criticisms noted above, we still believe that the application of PET technology to psychiatry has its brightest moments ahead. This is because we are dealing with a biochemical tool which is limited mainly by the ingenuity of the practitioners and their skill at isolating a particular brain function in an experimental paradigm. It is already clear that studies to date have consistently shown that regional energy metabolism in schizophrenics differs from that of normal controls. The criticisms raised in this review reflect the early difficulties expected when applying a complex technology to a poorly understood probably heretogeneous psychiatric syndrome. A high yield of direct evidence for central biochemical derangements in schizophrenia has been obtained from relatively few subjects. The development of positron labelled neuroreceptor ligands, transport markers, and the application of *in vivo* tracer kinetics to measure membrane properties in addition to the use of functional and pharmacological probes and test/retest strategies to complement the glucose and oxygen utilization studies promise a wealth of interpretable new information. The use of larger and better defined psychiatric populations with longitudinal studies on the one hand, and refined strategies for image analysis on the other, should lead to a delineation of the pathophysiology of schizophrenia and the other major psychiatric syndromes, a task for which PET is uniquely suited.

REFERENCES

American Psychiatric Association (1980). *Diagnostic and statistical manual of mental disorders* (3rd edn) (DSM III). Washington D.C.
Berner, P., Gabriel, E., Katschnig, H., Kieffer, W., Koehler, K., Lenz, GT., and Simhandl, C. (1983). *Diagnostic criteria for schizophrenic and affective psychoses.* World Psychiatric Association, Geneva.
Brodie, J. D., Christman, D. R., Corona, J. F., Fowley, J. S., Gomez-Mont, F., Jaeger, J., Michaels, P. A., Rotrosan, J., Russell, J. A., Volkos, N. D., Wikler, A., Wolf, A. P., and Wolkin, A. (1984). Patterns of metabolic activity in the treatment of schizophrenia. *Ann. Neurol.* **15** (Suppl), S166–S169.
Buchsbaum, M. S., Ingvar, D. H., Kessler, R. Waters, R. M., Cappeletti, J., Von Kammen, D. P., King, A. C., Johnson, J. L., Manning, R. G., Flynn, R. W., Mann, L. S., Burney, W. E., and Sokoloff, L. (1982). Cerebral glucography with positron tomography. *Arch. Gen. Psychiat.* **39**, 251–9.
Budinger, T. F., Deønzo, S. E., and Huesman, R. H. (1984). Instrumentation for positron emission tomography. *Ann. Neurol.* **15** (Suppl), S35–43.
Clark, C. M., Kessler, R., Buchsbaum, M. S., Margolin, R. A. and Holcomb, H. H.

(1984). Correlational methods for determining regional coupling of cerebral glucose metabolism: pilot study. *Biol. Psychiat.* **19**, 663–78.

DeChiro, G., Brooks, R. A., Patronas, N. J., Bairamian, D., Kornblith, P. L., Smith, B. H., Mangi, L. and Barker, J. (1984). Issues in the *in vivo* measurement of glucose metabolism of human central nervous system tumors. *Ann. Neurol.* **15** (Suppl), S138–S146.

Farkas, T., Reivich, M., Alavi, A., Greenberg, J. H., Fowler, J. S., MacGregor, R. R., Christman, D. R., and Wolf, A. P. (1980). The application of (18 F) fluorodeoxyglucose and positron emission tomography in the study of psychiatric conditions. In *Cerebral metabolism and neural function* (ed. J. V. Passonneau). Williams and Wilkins Co., Baltimore.

—— Wolf, A. P., Jaeger, J., Brodie, J., Christman, D., and Fowler, J. (1984). Regional brain glucose metabolism in chronic schizophrenia. *Arch. Gen. Psychiat.* **41**, 293–300.

Feighner, J. P., Robins, E., Guze, S. B., Woodruff, F. A., Winokur, G., and Munoz, R. (1972). Diagnostic criteria for use in psychiatric research. *Arch. Gen. Psychiat.* **26**, 57–63.

Feinstein, A. R. (1977). *Clinical biostatistics.* CV Mosby Co., St. Louis.

Fischer, R. A. (19660 *The design of experiments* (8th edn). Hafner Publishing Co., New York.

Frackowiak, R. S. J., Lenzi, GT. L., Jones, T., and Heather, J. D. (1980). Quantitative measurement of regional cerebral blood flow and oxygen metabolism in man using ^{15}O and positron emission tomography theory, procedure and normal values. *J. Comput. Assist. Tomogr.* **4**, 727–36.

Huang, S. C., Phelps, M. E., Hoffman, E. J., Sideris, K., Selin, C. J. and Kuhl, D. E. (1980). Non-invasive determination of local cerebral metabolic rate of glucose in man. *Am. J. Physiol.* **238**, E69–E82.

Ingvar, D. H. and Franzen, G. (1974). Abnormalities of cerebral blood flow distribution in patients with chronic schizophrenia. *Acta Psychiat. Scand.* **50**, 425–62.

Kety, S. S. and Schmidt, C. F. (1948). The nitrous oxide method for the quantitative determination of cerebral blood flow in man: theory, procedure and normal values. *J. Clin. Invest.* **27**, 476–82.

Lassen, N. A. and Ingvar, D. H. (1974). Radioisotopic assessment of regional cerebral blood flow. *Prog. Nucl. Med.* **2**, 1484–6.

Mazziotta, J. C. and Phelps, M. E. (1984). Human sensory stimulation and deprivation: positron emission tomographic results and strategies. *Ann. Neurol.* **15** (Supl), S50NS60.

—— Phelps, M. E., Halgren, E. (1983). Local cerebral glucose metabolic responses to audiovisual stimulation and deprivation: studies in human subjects with positron CT. *Hum. Neurobiol.* **2**, 11–23.

Overall, J. E. and Hollister, L. E. (1979). Comparative evaluation of research diagnostic criteria for schizophrenia. *Arch. Gen. Psychiat.* **36**, 1198–205.

Sacks, W., Sacks, S., and Fleischer, D. (1983). A comparison of the cerebral uptake and metabolism of labelled glucose and deoxyglucose *in vivo* in rats. *Neurochem Res.* **8**, 661–85.

Schneider, K. (1959). *Clinical psychopathology* (translated from 3rd edn by M. W. Hamilton and E. W. Anderson). Grune and Stratton, New York.

Sheppard, G., Gruzelier, J., Manchanda, R., Hirsch, S. R., Wise, R., Frackowiak, R. and Jones, T. (1983). 15-Oxygen positron emission tomographic scanning in predominantly never-treated acute schizophrenic patients. *Lancet.* **22(8365–66)**, 1448–52.

Sokoloff, L. (1981). Circulation and energy metabolism of the brain. In *Basic neurochemistry* (eds. G. J. Siegel, R. W. Albers, B. W. Agranoff and R. Katzman) pp. 471–493. Little, Brown and Co., Boston.

Spitzer, R. L., Endicott, J., and Robins, E. (1978*a*). *Research diagnostic criteria (RDC) for a selected group of functional disorders* (3rd edn). New York State Psychiatric Institute.
—— —— and —— (1978*b*). Research diagnostic criteria: rationale and reliability. *Arch. Gen. Psychiatr.* **35**, 773–82.
Widen, L. Bergstrom, M., Blomqvist, G., Brismar, T., Ehrim, E., Elander, S., Ericson, K., Eriksson, L., Greitz, T., Litton, J. E., Malmborg, T., Nilsson, L., Sedvall, G., and Ugglas, M. (1981). Glucose metabolism in patients with schizophrenia: emission computed tomography measurements with 11-C-glucose. *J. Cereb. Blood Flow Metab.* **1** (*Suppl* **1**); 455–6.
—— Blomqvist, G., Greitz, T., Litton, J. E., Bergstrom, M., Ehrim, E., Ericson, K., Eriksson, L., Ingvar, D. H., Johansson, L., Nilsson, J. L. G., Stone-Elander, S., Sedvall, G., Wiesel, F.,and Wiik, G. (1983). PET studies of glucose metabolism in patients with schizophrenia. *Am. J. Neuroradiol.* **4** , 550–2.
Wolkin, A., Jaeger,J., Brodie, J. D., Wolf, A. P., Fowler, J., Rotrosen, J., Gomez-Mont, F., and Cancro, R. (1985). Persistance of cerebral metabolic abnormalities in chronic schizophrenia as determined by P.E.T. *Am. J. Psychiat.* **142** 564–71.

ACKNOWLEDGEMENTS

Supported in part by Grant NS 15638 from the National Institute of Communicative Disorders and Stroke. The authors are indebted to their many colleagues at Brookhaven National Laboratory and New York University Medical Center. In particular, the unflagging interest and support of Dr Alfred Wolf in the application of PET to an understanding of schizophrenia is gratefully appreciated.

4

Positron emission tomography (PET) of regional cerebral glucose use in psychiatric patients

LYNN E. DELISI AND MONTE S. BUCHSBAUM

INTRODUCTION

Several hypotheses for the pathogenesis of major psychiatric disorders suggest abnormalities in specific regions of the brain, particularly frontal and temporal cortex, and the subcortical limbic and striatal structures.

Studies of subjects with defined lesions of the frontal lobe have linked symptoms of emotional inappropriateness or lability, avolition, flat affect, and social incompetence to this area of the brain (Benson and Blumer 1975; Luria 1966), while studies of patients with lesions of the temporal cortex, particularly the left, have shown an association of this region with alterations in auditory and visual integration, and language communication and organization (Penfield 1954; Hillbom 1980). These are all aspects of behaviour found to be abnormal in schizophrenic and affective disorders, although the clusters and predominance of symptoms vary.

In addition, biochemical hypotheses of altered dopaminergic activity, as well as that of other related neuroregulators in these disorders suggest that the structures of the limbic system and striatum (the regions of the brain rich in dopaminergic neurons) are also of particular interest (DeLisi and Wyatt 1984). Some data from post-mortem pathological and biochemical studies are consistent with these hypotheses, although there are inconsistencies in the literature that remain to be resolved (Reynolds *et al.* 1983; Crow *et al.* 1982; Farley *et al.* 1980; Stevens 1982; Bogerts *et al.* 1983; Brown *et al.* 1984).

Position emission tomography (PET) is a newly developed technique to quantify regional brain metabolism *in vivo* in humans, and thus may aid in clarifying the above hypothesized local changes. For a review of the methodology, see Phelps *et al.* (1982) and *The Annals of Neurology Supplement* **15**, 1984. While clinical utility has been established for the use of this procedure for the diagnosis of cancer and certain neurological diseases, the studies of psychiatric patients have not resulted in new evidence at present that demonstrate specific regional metabolic alterations. There have been some interesting findings, however, the significance of which are presently unclear.

Several independent investigative groups have now reported a decrease in frontal metabolic activity relative to posterior cortical brain activity in chronic schizophrenic patients compared with controls (Buchsbaum *et al.* 1982; Widen *et al.* 1983; Farkas *et al.* 1984). These studies are consistent with the earlier work of Ingvar and Franzen (1974) using labelled xenon carotid artery injections for the measurement of cerebral blood flow. They reported a relationship of decreased frontal blood flow in older chronic schizophrenic patients with the degree of overall psychopathology and the severity of catatonic symptoms and withdrawal, while increased occipito/ temporal flow was correlated with the severity of disorganization of thought processes. Since cerebral blood flow is assumed from animal studies to be correlated with glucose use, it is of interest that the phenomenon of 'hypo-frontality' in schizophrenic patients, as coined by Ingvar and Franzen, has been at least partially confirmed in other more recent blood flow studies (Ariel *et al.* 1983; Berman *et al.* 1984). Not all investigators have replicated this finding, however (Gur *et al.* 1983; Gur and Gur 1984; Kety *et al.* 1948; Gordon *et al.* 1955; Hoyer and Oesterreich 1975; Mathew *et al.* 1982).

One difficulty in interpretation of many of the PET and blood flow studies is that most patients with major psychiatric disorders have been chronically medicated, and the effects of anti-depressant and anti-psychotic pharma-cological agents on overall and regional brain metabolism have not been established. One study using oxygen-15 metabolism with PET (Sheppard *et al.* 1983), another method that measures both cerebral blood flow and metabolic rates, found no differences in metabolic gradients in young first-episode schizophrenic patients, who, for the most part, had never been treated with neuroleptic medication. A second study of 13 largely first-episode schizophrenics, using [^{11}C]deoxyglucose, also failed to find evidence of hypofrontality in these patients, but rather found an increase in the frontal/ posterior ratio due to decreased parietal activity (Widen *et al.* 1984). While the results of these studies suggest that hypofrontality may develop after the onset of the illness and be either a result of chronicity or the pharmacological treatment of the disorder, several problems with the methods used prevent the establishment of any definitive conclusions. Table 4.1 summarizes the numerous factors that can contribute to artifactual results obtained from PET. A few to emphasize include: the wide variation in gradients that may exist when the conditions during the scan procedure are not controlled and the subject is only at rest, and the importance of the height of the scan section used for analyses [i.e. Buchsbaum *et al.* (1982) found maximal hypofrontality in a supraventricular slice, while other studies may have used lower brain slices only for analyses, or fail to describe which one is used (Georgotas 1984)]. In addition, the data in the Sheppard *et al.* (1983) study shows greater oxygen metabolism in posterior relative to frontal regions in not only the schizophrenics, but normal controls as well; that is, the frontal/posterior ratios are signficantly lower than those found by investigators using labelled glucose, suggesting that studies using oxygen as a tracer may not be compar-

TABLE 4.1. *Sources of potential artifacts related to final PET results.*

Compound used as tracer
  1. Half-life and breakdown rate of label
  2. Purity of compound
  3. Differences in oxygen vs glucose
  4. Differences in positron-emitting labels (i.e. 18_F vs 11_C)

Experimental conditions
  1. Variation in anxiety and emotional state of normal subjects
  2. Psychiatric state of patient (agitation, movements, distractibility)
  3. Task performed during uptake
  4. Variation in eye/ear closures, as well as other sensory inputs
  5. Prolonged uptake period and thus inconsistent physiological changes
  6. Variation in blood-sampling procedures (arterial vs venous blood, etc.)
  7. Failure to control for gender and age differences

PET
  1. Limited resolution (spatial and temporal)
  2. Non-uniform resolution
  3. Scatter and partial volume effects
  4. Inadequate number of planes for anatomic sampling
  5. Need to standardize adequately to phantoms
  6. Inability to standardize planes among individuals due to variation in head size and shapes
  7. Movement of head in scanner
  8. Change in distribution of tracer compound during scan procedure from first to last slice

Data analysis
  1. Inaccuracy of models to describe biochemical kinetics
  2. No appropriate model for substances studied
  3. Relating kinetic constants derived in animals to human studies
  4. Difference in kinetics between white and grey matter
  5. Difficulty in matching same slices among individuals
  6. Undersampling of anatomical structures
  7. Overinterpretation of assumed anatomical details
  8. Computerized methods do not account for anatomical differences among individuals
  9. Accounting for cortical folding
 10. Lack of serial determinations of data in same individual over time to obtain normal variation

---

able to the deoxyglucose studies. Finally, with regard to the PET studies completed with the use of labelled 2-deoxyglucose (2-DG) uptake into the brain cells as a measure of overall metabolism of these cells, not only is the principle behind this model controversial (Fox 1984), but this compound is not selective for cells producing specific neurotransmitters or regulators. Since abnormalities in the metabolism of only one or a small number of neurochemicals may be related to schizophrenia or the major affective disorders, the future use of specific ligands with PET, such as the dopamine agonists or antagonists (Wager *et al.* 1983) that bind to specific neuronal receptors, will enable investigators to clarify the roles of these neurochemicals in mentation and disease processes, as well as their relationship to the overall metabolic patterns already described.

  In addition to the above problems it is worth noting the results of PET and blood flow studies of other psychiatric and related neurological disorders, although some of these have been less extensive. The hypofrontal pattern described in chronic schizophrenic patients has also been found in patients with affective disorder (Buchsbaum *et al.* 1985), although the studies of affective disorder conflict, and may depend on clinical subdiagnosis (i.e. unipolar or bipolar) and mental state during the procedure (Phelps *et al.* 1984). In organic dementias, however, blood flow studies have shown an overall reduction in total blood flow that is proportional to the intellectual defect (Freyhan *et al.* 1951; Lassen *et al.* 1960). Alzheimer's dementia patients have specific reductions in parietal cortex that actually result in what appears to be relatively elevated frontal to posterior gradients (Chase *et al.* 1984). In other studies, adults who were diagnosed as childhood autism had increased overall metabolic activity (Rumsey *et al.* 1985), as did adult subjects with mongolism (Schwartz *et al.* 1983).

Few PET studies have been reported on patients with Parkinson's disease, a disorder thought to result from loss of dopaminergic neurons in the substantia nigra and thus decreased dopamine concentrations. While global cerebral metabolism appears decreased in Parkinsonian patients from one study (Kuhl *et al.* 1984), the relative distribution of glucose throughout the brain remains normal. Patients with Huntington's disease, on the other hand, were found to have decreased glucose utilization in the caudate and putamen, while metabolism appeared normal throughout the rest of the brain (Kuhl *et al.* 1984). The Parkinson's patients in these studies were all receiving L-dopa, while the majority of the Huntington's chorea patients were medicated with neuroleptics.

While caution is needed in directly applying the results from quantitative radioautographic animal studies to human physiology and the PET studies, nevertheless, some interesting parallels exist that may help in the interpretation of some of these findings. For example, both acute and chronic doses of amphetamine have been administered to animals followed by the quantification of local cerebral glucose metabolism. Amphetamine can produce marked behavioural changes in animals and a paranoid psychosis sometimes indistinguishable from paranoid schizophrenia in humans. Its mechanism of action is thought to be through decreasing the normal synaptic uptake of catecholamines, particularly dopamine. Acute doses of amphetamine to rats were found to stimulate glucose utilization in several cerebral structures, particularly those of the extrapyramidal motor system, while there appeared to be no effects in mesolimbic regions. More sustained chronic administration, however, resulted in a specific increase in the nucleus accumbens, an impotant structure of the mesolimbic system, and one rich in catecholamine concentrations (Orzi *et al.* 1983). It should be noted that the animal studies do not suggest changes in cortical gradients of activity with pharmacological manipulation, and the PET studies in humans at present lack the resolution necessary to look for the localized alterations seen in animal studies.

Some of the medications used for long-term treatment of psychiatric disorders have also been studied using the deoxyglucose technique in rats. In one study (Gerber *et al.* 1983) desmethylimipramine (DMI), a tricyclic antidepressant, was found to increase glucose utilization in 11 brain regions acutely, while chronic administration decreased glucose use in seven of 30 brain regions. The regions affected included those of the occipital cortex, thalamus, limbic system, striatum, and hypothalamus. Phenelzine, a monoamine oxidase inhibitor, on the other hand, had relatively little effect on glucose utilization given either in acute or chronic doses. In another study (McCulloch *et al.* 1982), the anti-psychotic, haloperidol, administered in acute doses to rats decreased glucose utilization in the majority of brain regions, while specifically increasing glucose utilization in the nucleus accumbens. Taken together, these studies are important references for interpreting the human PET studies of patients with major psychiatric disorders, although they have not clarified many of the unresolved issues, and point to the difficulty in extrapolating from animal to human studies.

The following report reviews the series of PET studies of chronic medication-free schizophrenic and affective disorder patients performed at the National Institute of Mental Health, Bethesda, Maryland, and examines the effect of neuroleptic medication on glucose metabolism in a subgroup of nine of the schizophrenic patients (Buchsbaum *et al.* 1982, 1984; Delisi *et al.* 1985*a*, *b*).

METHODS

Study 1

The following is a summary of the subjects and methods of the initial PET study, details of which are reported elsewhere (Buchsbaum *et al.* 1982).

Eight DSM-III-diagnosed chronic schizophrenic patients (six males and two females), who were medication-free for at least 2 weeks and hospitalized on a National Institute of Health research unit at the time of scan, were compared with six normal volunteers (four males and two females). All subjects were in the resting state during the glucose-absorption period.

For data analyses, slices were identified and matched by anatomical landmarks. For each slice, the outer brain contour was outlined with a boundary-finding technique developed for the skull on CT scans. The outline-positioning criteria was 50 per cent of the highest mean level observed in an appropriate 1-cm square block of cortex. A vertical meridian was computed by fitting a straight line using least-squares fit to the midpoints of a series of horizontal lines that connected the left and right sides of the slice outline. An analysis of the outer rim of the brain (mainly cortex) was done by peeling a 2.3 cm radial strip for quantification of glucose use. This peel was further subdivided into two segments for each quadrant and the activity was expressed in ratios of sectors to mean whole-slice activities, as well as anterior/posterior gradients (top left plus right frontal sectors over left plus right upper occipital sectors; see Fig. 4.1).

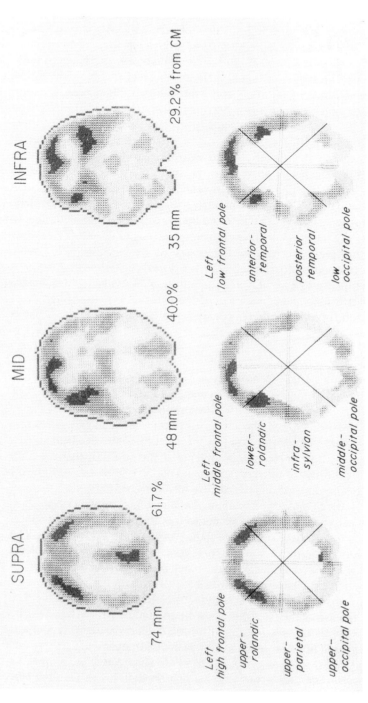

Fig. 4.1. Demonstration of the peel analysis method. PET image is outlined by a boundary-finding algorithm (top images), and vertical and hor-izontal meridians are fitted by the least-squares method. Next, a radial scan from their intersection defines a 2.3 cm-thick peel, which is divided into four sectors in each hemisphere. Anterior/posterior gradients are obtained for the supraslice using a ratio of the left plus right top frontal sectors to the left plus right upper occipital sectors.

Study 2

Twenty-one DSM-III-diagnosed chronic schizophrenic patients (15 males and six females, mean age (± S.D.) OF 28 (± 7), range 18–51), 20 DSM-III-diagnosed major depressive disorder patients (eight males and 12 females, mean age (± S.D.) of 38.7 (± 12), range 24–60), and 21 age- and gender-matched normal controls (15 males and six females, 32 (± 11 years of age) participated in the PET procedure described above and in more detail elsewhere (Buchsbaum *et al.* 1985). The schizophrenic patients were recruited from four independent schizophrenia research programs: The Biological Psychiatry Branch (*n*=4); The Clinical Neuroscience Branch, NIMH, Bethesda, Maryland (*n*=6); The Adult Psychiatry Branch, NIMH, St. Elizabeths Hospital, Washington, D.C., (*n*=6); The Maryland Psychiatric Research Center, University of Maryland School of Medicine, Catonsville, Maryland (*n*=5). These centres consisted of three independent units of predominantly psychotic inpatients and a group of relatively stable, but chronic, outpatients respectively. Two patients were referred by private outpatient psychiatrists. All patients were medication-free for at least 2 weeks prior to the scan [mean of 29.3 (± 28) days]. These patients did not overlap with the Study 1 sample. The depressed patients were also recruited from three independent NIMH research units: The Biological Psychiatry Branch (*n*=13); The Neuropharmacology Branch (*n*=4); The Psychogenetic Outpatient Section (*n*=3). Depressed patients were medication-free for a minimum of 2 weeks [mean 33.4 (± 29) days].

The controls were recruited from the surrounding community and were without any medical disorders, alcohol or drug abuse, or history of psychiatric illness in self or a first-degree relative.

Patients were diagnosed and subtyped according to DSM-III criteria by the primary psychiatrist responsible for each patient's care. An additional pre-scan screening evaluation was done on all patients using material from semi-structured interviews with the patients, chart review, and discussions with primary-care staff. An NIMH-modified version of the brief psychiatric rating scale (BRPS; Overall and Gorham 1963) was completed on 20 of the schizophrenic patients during the scan procedure. Scores range from 26 to a maximum pathology score of 182. Depression on the day of the scan of the affective disorder patients was rated using the Bunney–Hamburg psychosis scale (1963; score range 1–10).

Anxiety during the scan procedure was scored for all controls using the Spielberger anxiety scale (Spielberger *et al.* 1970).

The procedure was the same as in Study 1, with the following changes: During the period of absorption, subjects were receiving somatosensory stimulation to the right forearm. This consisted of 1/s single, 1 ms biphasic square-wave constant-current shocks of four intensities, ranging from barely perceptible (2 mA) to unpleasant (23 mA) presented in a random order. Pain stimulation was chosen as the sensory condition because of its known frontal activation and differential responsiveness in schizophrenia. In addition, constant-current cutaneous electrical stimulation is highly reproducible, can be administered for 30 min, and does not depend on eye fixation, or other peripheral factors associated with visual stimulation.

Similar analyses of the data were also performed. Anterior/posterior gradients and mean cortical glucose use were calculated on the lowest slice above the lateral ventricles that clearly showed midline cortical grey matter and the largest cortical rim. This is the slice that in Study 1 was found to show the largest differences between schizophrenics and controls. Basal ganglia activity was calculated for the midventricular slice, the slice that most clearly shows the lateral ventricles and underlying striatum. Pixel boxes (4×4) were visually placed symmetrically under each lateral ventricle using an atlas derived computer program. Temporal lobe analyses were performed on the infra-slice, the first slice below the lateral ventricles that include part of the third ventricle and cerebellum according to matched atlas sections (Matsui and Hirano 1978) and the peel analyses were performed using the sectors that correspond to anterior and posterior temporal cortex. Inferior temporal lobes were also analysed using a boundary-finding algorithm to outline the temporal lobes in the most posterior slice (approximately 18 mm above the canthomeatal line). Cerebellar activity was also outlined by the above technique and quantified in the most posterior slice (DeLisi *et al.* 1985*c*).

Study 3

Eight of the patients from Study 2 and one patient from Study 1 returned for a follow-up PET scan, under the same conditions of the original scan, when they were stabilized on a dose of neuroleptic medication titrated to produce a maximum clinical response. Four patients were medicated with fluphenazine, two with haloperidol, one with chlorpromazine, one with thioridizine, and one with loxapine. The patients were medicated from 36 days to 32 months (mean of 7.4 months) prior to the repeat scan. All conditions for the procedure were standardized within individuals and scan slices were matched to obtain identical levels for each slice obtained. Analyses were performed on each scan in a similar manner to those for Study 2. This study is described in more detail in DeLisi *et al.* (1985*a*).

RESULTS

There were no differences in mean cortical glucose use for subjects and controls from either Study 1 or 2. Females in Study 2 tended to have higher overall glucose use than males (normals: 22.8 ± 8 vs 19.2 ± 6; schizophrenics: 24.5 ± 4 vs 22.7 5), but this difference did not reach statistical significance. Anxiety in the normal controls as rated by the Spielberger anxiety scale tended to correlate inversely with the amount of glucose use (pearson $r = -54$; $P = 0.06$). There was no evidence of hemispheric laterality in glucose use in either patient or control groups. See Table 4.2 for cortical glucose use comparisons. For both the schizophrenic and affective disorder patients, the

TABLE 4.2. *Glucose use ($\mu mol\ 100\ g^{-1}\ min^{-1}$).*

Subjects	Anterior/posterior gradient	Max. temporal cortex glucose use		Mean caudate glucose use		Maximum cerebellar glucose use
		Left	Right	Left	Right	
Chronic schizophrenics medication-free at rest ($n = 8$)	$1.06 \pm 0.06^*$	19.1 ± 7.5	20.4 ± 7.8			21.6 ± 5.1
Normal controls at rest ($n = 6$)	1.12 ± 0.05	13.2 ± 6.4	14.3 ± 6.2			17.6 ± 9.0
Chronic schizophrenics medication-free somatosensory stimulation ($n = 21$)	$1.04 \pm 0.09^*$	$19.5 \pm 3.8^*$	$18.7 \pm 3.8^*$	24.8 ± 5.7 ($n = 9$)	24.6 ± 6.1 ($n = 9$)	$18.7 \pm 4.4^*$ ($n = 14$)
Normal controls somatosensory stimulation ($n = 21$)	1.11 ± 0.10	14.8 ± 4.4	15.1 ± 4.7	29.0 ± 6.8 ($n = 16$)	29.3 ± 7.4 ($n = 16$)	14.9 ± 3.9 ($n = 18$)
Affective disorders medication-free somatosensory stimulation ($n = 20$)	$1.02 \pm 0.09^*$ ($n = 11$)	$19.2 \pm 5.2^*$	17.0 ± 4.3			$19.9 \pm 4.5^*$ ($n = 11$)

* $P < 0.05$ (2-tailed *t*-test).

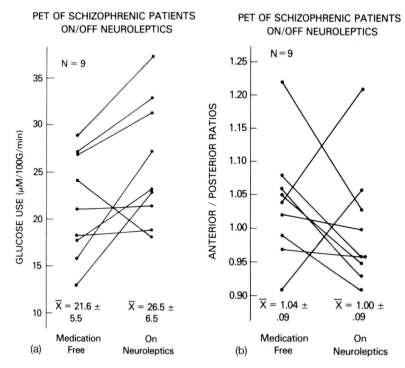

Fig. 4.2(a). Mean cortical glucose use for nine chronic schizophrenic patients on and off neuroleptic medication (paired *t*-test, *t* = 2.6, *P* = 0.02). (b) Anterior/posterior gradients for nine chronic chizophrenic patients on and off neuroleptic medication (paired *t*-test, *t* = 0.92, N.S.).

time medication-free was not significantly correlated with anterior/posterior ratios. There was, however, a significant increase in cortical glucose use in the nine patients in the medicated state (see Fig. 4.2a).

Anterior/posterior gradients were significantly different compared with controls for schizophrenic patients in Study 1 and both patient groups in Study 2 (see Table 4.2). The amount of decline in this gradient failed to correlate with degree of psychopathology, as defined by overall BPRS ratings, BPRS symptom clusters, and most individual BPRS items. There were only 4 of 26 significant correlations (pearson *r*): emotional withdrawal (*r* = 0.59), disorientation (*r* = 0.520), distractibility (*r* = 0.51), and helplessness/hopelessness (*r* = 0.48) and these were in the schizophrenic patients in a direction opposite to that expected. In the depressed patients, degree of depression did not correlate with anterior/posterior ratios. There was no significant change in the gradient in the nine patients repeated in the medicated state, despite overall improvement in clinical state with medication in the majority of these patients (see Fig. 4.2b).

Glucose use in the striatum was not significantly different in the patient groups compared with controls; the nine patients when medicated, however,

TABLE 4.3. *Glucose use (μmol 100 g⁻¹ min⁻¹).*

	Patients (n = 9)		paired	
	Medication-free	Medicated	t	P
Caudate glucose use				
Left mean	24.8 ± 5.7	32.7 ± 7.8	2.79	< 0.02
Right mean	24.6 ± 6.1	32.9 ± 8.9	2.65	< 0.02
Left mean/slice mean	1.21 ± 0.12	1.33 ± 0.18	2.01	< 0.10
Right mean/slice mean	1.16 ± 0.17	1.32 ± 0.15	2.24	< 0.05
Temporal cortex glucose use				
Left maximum	19.1 ± 3.4	22.5 ± 3.7	3.15	< 0.01
Right maximum	18.9 ± 4.1	21.1 ± 3.9	1.61	
Left maximum/slice maximum	0.82 ± 0.11	0.93 ± 0.12	0.39	
Right maximum/slice maximum	0.80 ± 0.08	0.78 ± 0.13	0.35	
Left/right maximum	1.02 ± 0.08	1.07 ± 0.06	1.32	

had significant increases in striatal glucose use (see Table 4.3) that were then statistically elevated over normal control values.

Temporal cortex activity was increased in both schizophrenic (Study 1 and 2) and affective disorder patients compared with controls in both slice levels analysed. This difference appeared to be greater on the left in the schizophrenics and depressed patients. These differences, however, were even further magnified in the schizophrenic patients on medication (see Table 4.3). While temporal cortex glucose activity was not correlated with BPRS measures of psychopathology for the schizophrenic patients, the degree of depression was associated with greater relative temporal activity in the affective disorder patients.

Increased cerebellar activity was also noted in both groups of patients compared with controls. (Table 4.2).

DISCUSSION

Studies of overall brain metabolism using PET have resulted in a series of differences between patients with major psychiatric disorders and normal healthy volunteers. A decrease in the normal hyperfrontal distribution of metabolic activity has been found; however it is not specific to one clinical entity, has not been found to be present in acute patients near the onset of their illness, is not changed with treatment, and does not appear to be relevant to any of the hypotheses of aetiology of these conditions.

Overall metabolic activity is less specific, since it appears to be altered by changes in the normal emotional state (i.e. anxiety) and may be influenced by gender, medications, and decline with age and intellectual functioning. In addition, artifactual variables, i.e. such as differences in calculations, blood clearance, the injectable compound, and day to day variation in the physical apparatus have to be considered.

We have confirmed other PET and blood flow studies finding the presence of a hypofrontal metabolic distribution in schizophrenic patients at rest and under conditions to stimulate the frontal lobe. The meaning of this change, which is only about a 10 per cent difference in activity, remains uncertain. Post-mortem pathological changes have been localized to structures of the limbic system, and have not been noted in frontal or occipital lobes. The absolute metabolic activity of patients in specific subcortical limbic structures were not available to us, given the limited resolution of our scanner.

The increased activity in the temporal lobes bilaterally is of notable interest, though it is not known what specific neuronal activity is increased as a result. Brodie and associates (see Chapter 3), on the other hand, find decreased temporal lobe activity in schizophrenics which normalizes with treatment. This finding is consistent with the findings in temporal lobe epileptics (see Trimble, Chapter 6) of decreased left temporal activity in those patients with psychosis and epilepsy.

striatal activity does not appear different between patients and controls, but is increased in patients medicated with neuroleptics, is lack of support for a hyperdopaminergic system in schizophrenia, but, nevertheless, supports the effect that neuroleptics act on dopamine-rich neurons.

Since all these variables seem even further deviated from normal with medication and improvement in mental status, these results suggest a lack of a direct correlation of these changes with the disease pathology. Furthermore, these data may indicate that a minimum of 2 weeks is not a long enough medication-free period for such studies.

REFERENCES

Ariel, R. N., Golden, C. J., Berg, R. A., Quaife, M. A., Dirksen, J. W., Forsell, T., Wilson, J., and Graber, B. (1983). Regional cerebral blood flow in schizophrenics: Tests using the xenon (Xe-133) inhalation method. *Arch. Gen. Psychiat.* **40**, 258–63.

Benson, F. and Blumer, D. (1975). *Psychiatric aspects of neurological disease.* Grune and Stratton, New York.

Berman, K. F., Zec, R. F., and Weinberger, D. R. (1984). Impaired frontal cortical function in schizophrenia. rCBR evidence. *Abstracts of the Annual Meeting of the Society of Biological Psychiatry, Los Angeles, California*, p. 60.

Bogerts, B., Hantsch, J., and Herzer, M. A. (1983). Morphometric study of the dopamine-containing cell groups in the mesencephalon of normals, parkinson patients and schizophrenics. *Biol. Psychiat.* **18**, 951–70.

Brown, R., Colter, N., Corsellis, J. A. N., Crow, T. J., Frith, C. D., Jagoe, R., Johnstone, E. C., and Mash, L. (1984). Changes in brain weight and structure in the functional psychoses. *2nd Biannual Winter Workshop on Schizophrenia, Davos, Switzerland.*

Buchsbaum, M. S., Ingvar, D. H., Kessler, R., Waters, R. N., Cappelletti, J., van Kammen, D. P., King, A. C., Johnson, J. L., Manning, R. G., Flynn, R. W., Mann, L. S., Bunney, W. E., and Sokoloff, L. (1982). Cerebral glucography with positron tomography. *Arch. Gen. Psychiat.* **39**, 251–9.

—— DeLisi, L. E., Holcomb, H. H., Cappelletti, J., King, A. C., Johnson, J., Hazlett, E., Dowling-Zimerman, S., Post, R. M., Morihisa, J., Carpenter, W., Cohen, R., Pickar, D., Weinberger, D. R., Margolin, R., and Kessler, R. M. (1984). Anteroposterior gradients in cerebral glucose use in schizophrenia and affective disorders. *Arch. Gen. Psychiat.* **41**, 1159–68.

Bunney, W. E., Jr., and Hamburg, D. A. (1963). Methods for reliable longitudinal observation of behavior. *Arch. Gen. Psychiat.* **9**, 280–94.

Chase, T. N., Foster, N. L., Fedio, P., Brooks, R., Mansi, L., and DiChiro, G. (1984). Regional cortical dysfunction in Alzheimer's disease as determined by positron emission tomography. *Ann. Neurol.* **15** (*suppl.*), S170–S174.

Crow, T. J., Cross, A. J., Johnstone, E. C., and Owen, F. (1982). Two syndromes in schizophrenia and their pathogenesis. In *Schizophrenia as a brain disease*, (eds H. A. Nasrallah and F. A. Henn) pp. 196–234. Oxford University Press, Oxford.

DeLisi, L. E. and Wyatt, R. J. (1984). Neurochemical aspects of schizophrenia. In *Handbook of neurochemistry* (ed. A. Lajtha) Vol. 10. Plenum, New York.

—— Holcomb, H. H., Cohen, R. M., Pickar, D., Carpenter, W., Morihisa, J. M., King, A. C., Kessler, R., Margolin, R., and Buchsbaum, M. S. (1985*a*). Positron emission tomography (PET) in schizophrenic patients with and without neuroleptic treatment. *J. Cereb. Blood Flow Metab.* **5**, 201–6.

—— Buchsbaum, M. S., Holcomb, H. H., Pickar, D., Boronow, J., Morihisa, J. M., van Kammen, D. P., Carpenter, W., Kessler, R., Margolin, R., and Cohen, R. M. (1985*b*). Clinical correlates of decreased anterposterior gradients in positron emission tomography (PET) of schizophrenic patients. *Am. J. Psychiat.* **142**, 78–81.

—— Buchsbaum, M. S., Holcomb, H. H., Langston, K. C., King, A. C., Kessler, R., Pickar, D., Carpenter, W., Morihisa, J. M., Margolin, R., Weinberger, D. R., and Cohen, R. (1985*c*). Increased temporal lobe glucose use in chronic schizophrenic patients. *Biol. Psychiat.* (in press).

Farkas, T., Wolf, A. P., Jaeger, J., Brodie, J. D., Christman, D. R., and Fowler, J. S. (1984). Regional brain glucose metabolism in chronic schizophrenia. *Arch. Gen. Psychiat.* **41**, 293–300.

Farley, I. J., Sharnak, K. S., and Hornykiewicz, O. (1980). Brain monoamine changes in chronic paranoid schizophrenics and their possible relation to increased dopamine receptor sensitivity. In *Receptors for neurotransmitters and peptide hormones* 427–34. Raven Press, New York.

Fox, J. L. (1984). PET scan controversy aired. *Science* **224**, 143–4.

Freyhan, F. A., Woodford, R. B., and Kety, S. S. (1951). Cerebral blood flow and metabolism in psychoses of senility. *J. Nerv. Ment. Dis.* **113**, 449–56.

Georgotas, A. (1984). Positron emission tomography studies in affective disorders. *Clin. Neuropharmacol.* **7** (*Suppl.* **1**), 532–3.

Gerber, J. C., Choki, J., Brunswick, D. J., Reivich, M., and Frazer, A. (1983). The effect of antidepressant drugs on regional cerebral glucose utilization in the rat. *Brain Res.* **269**, 319–25.

Gordon, G. S., Estess, F. M., Adams, J. E., Bowman, K. M., and Simon, A. (1955). Cerebral oxygen uptake in chronic schizophrenic reaction. *Arch. Neurol. Psychiat.* (*Chic.*) **73**, 544–5.

Gur, R. E. and Gur, R. C. (1984). Regional cerebral blood flow in schizophrenics. *Clin. Neuropharmacol.* **7** (*Suppl.* **1**), 536–7.

—— Skolnick, B. E., Gur, R. C., Carof, S., Rieger, W., Obrist, W. D., Younkin, D., and Reivich, M. (1983). Brain function in psychiatric disorders: I. Regional cerebral blood flow in medicated schizophrenics. *Arch. Gen. Psychiat.* **40**, 1250–4.

Hillbom, E. (1980). Rehabilitation of veterans with cerebral injuries in Finland. *Diag. Med.* **32**, 1884–6.

Hoyer, S. and Oesterreich, K. (1975). Blood flow and oxidative metabolism of the brain in patients with schizophrenia. *Psychiat. Clin.* **8(6)**, 304–13.

Ingvar, D. H. and Franzen, G. (1974). Abnormalities of cerebral blood flow distribution in patients with chronic schizophrenia. *Acta Psychiat. Scand.* **50**, 425–62.

Kety, S. S., Woodford, R. B., Harmel, M. H., Freyhan, K. E., Appel, K. E., and Schmidt, C. F. (1948). Cerebral blood flow and metabolism in schizophrenia. *Am. J. Psychiat.* **104**, 765–70.

Kuhl, D. E., Metter, E. J., Riege, W. H., and Markham, C. H. (1984). Patterns of cerebral glucose utilization in Parkinson's disease and Huntington's disease. *Ann. Neurol.* **15** (*Suppl*), S119–S125.

Lassen, N. A., Feinberg, I., and Lane, M. H. (1960). Bilateral studies of cerebral oxygen uptake in young and aged normal subjects and in patients with organic dementia. *J. Clin. Invest.* **39**, 491–500.

Luria, A. R. (1966). *Higher cortical functions in man.* Basic Books, New York.

Mathew, R. J., Barr, D. L., Duncan, G. C., and Weinman, M. L. (1982). Regional cerebral blood flow in schizophrenia. *Arch. Gen. Psychiat.* **39**, 1121–4.

Matsui, T. and Hirano, A. (1978). *An atlas of the human brain for computerized tomography.* Igaku-Shoin, Tokyo.

McCulloch, J., Savaki, H. E., and Sokoloff, L. (1982). Distribution of effects of haloperidol on energy metabolism in the rat brain. *Brain Res.* **2443**, 81–90.

Orzi, F., Dow-Edwards, D., Jehle, J., Kenedy, C., and Sokoloff, L. (1983). Comparative effects of acute and chronic administration of amphetamine on local cerebral glucose utilization in the conscious rat. *J. Cereb. Blood Flow Metab.* **3**, 154–60.

Overall, J. E. and Gorham, D. R. (1963). *The brief psychiatric rating scale.* Psychol. Rep. 10: 799–812. NIHM Modification obtained from Dr L. Bigelow, William A. White Building, St. Elizabeths Hospital, Washington, D.C.

Penfield, W. (1954). Mechanisms of voluntary movement. *Brain* **77**, 1–17.

Phelps, M. E., Mazziotta, J. C., and Huang, S.-C. (1982). Review: study of cerebral function with positron computed tomography. *J. Cereb. Blood Flow Metab.* **2**, 113–62.

—— —— Baxter, L., and Gerner, R. (1984). Positron emission tomographic study of affective disorders: problems and strategies. *Ann. Neurol.* **15** (*Suppl*), S149–S156.

Reynolds, G. P. (1983). Increased concentrations and lateral asymmetry of amygdala dopamine in schizophrenia. *Nature, Lond.* **306**, 527–9.

Rumsey, J. M., Duara, R., Grady, C., Rapoport, J. L., Margolin, R. A., Rapoport, S. I., and Cutler, N. (1985). Brain metabolism in autism: resting cerebral glucose utilization as measured with positron emission tomography (PET). *Arch. Gen. Psychiat.* (in press).

Schwartz, M., Duara, R., Haxby, J., Grady, C., White, B. J., Kessler, r. M., Kay, A. D., Cutler, N. R., and Rapoport, S. I. (1983). Down's syndrome in adults: brain metabolism. *Science* **221**, 781–3.

Sheppard, G., Gruzelier, J., Manchanda, R., Hirsch, S. R., Wise, R., Frackowiak, R., and Jones, T. (1983). 15-O Positron emission tomographic scanning in predominantly never-treated acute schizophrenic patients. *Lancet* **ii**, 1448–52.

Spielberger, C. D., Gorsuch, R. L., and Luschene, R. E. (1970). *Manual for the state-trait anxiety inventory* Consulting Psychologist Press, Palo Alto, California.

Stevens, J. (1982). Neuropathology of schizophrenia. *Arch. Gen. Psychiat.* **39**, 1131–9.

Wagner, H. N., Burns, H. D., Dannals, R. F., Wong, D. F., Langstrom, B., Duelfer, T., Frost, J. J., Ravert, H. T., Links, J. M., Rosenblom, S. B., Lukas, S. E., Kramer, A. V., and Kuhar, M. J. (1983). Imaging dopamine receptors in the human brain by positron tomography. *Science* **221**, 1264–6.

Widen, L., Blomqvist, G., Greitz, T., Litton, J. E., Bergstrom, M., Ehrin, E., Ericson, K., Eriksson, L., Ingvar, D. H., Johansson, L., Nilsson, J. L., Stone-Elander, S., Sedvall, G., Wiesel, F., and Wiik, G. (1983). PET studies of glucose metabolism in patients with schizophrenia. *Am. J. Neurodiol.* **4**, 550–2.

—— —— De Paulis, T., Ehrin, E., Eriksson, L., Farde, L., Greitz, T., Hedstrom, C. G., Ingvar, D. H., Litton, J. E., Nilsson, J. L. G., Ogren, S. O., Sedvall, G., Stone-Elander, S., Wiesel, F.-A., and Wik, G. (1984). Studies of schizophrenia with positron CT. *Clin. Neuropharmacol.* **7** (*Suppl.* **1**), 548–9.

5

Pharmacokinetic studies using positron emission tomography

B. MAZIÈRE, D. COMAR, AND M. MAZIÈRE

INTRODUCTION

Positron emission tomography (PET), a non-invasive technique which allows the quantitative determination of tissue radioactivity in a living subject previously injected with a radiotracer has opened up possibilities of measurement of regional brain pharmacokinetics *in vivo* in humans (Ter-Pogossian *et al.* 1975; Phelps 1977).

This combined approach (i.e. intravenous administration of a compound labelled with a short-lived positron-emitting isotope and external detection of the radioactivity in transverse sections of the body) has at least two different applications in the pharmacokinetic field: (1) measurement of the fate of a labelled compound in 'normal' and diseased brain, i.e. penetration across the blood–brain barrier (BBB), distribution, equilibrium, biodegradation, and elimination (Comar *et al.* 1979; Baron *et al.* 1983; Ramsay 1983; Yamamoto *et al.* 1982); (2) use of a labelled compound as a radioligand to estimate the density, distribution, and function of specific binding sites (Mazière *et al.* 1982; Comar and Mazière 1982), the prime objective being to correlate the measured parameters with various physiological and pharmacological states or with clinically diagnosable disease states.

In this chapter we will illustrate these two applications of PET using some examples taken from various studies performed at the Service Hospitalier Frédéric Joliot.

REGIONAL PHARMACOKINETIC DETERMINATION

A study of 5, 5-diphenylhydantoin (DPH), a well-known anti-epileptic drug (Baron *et al.* 1983*a*) exemplifies the use of the PET technique for tissue pharmacokinetic determination.

DPH has for a long time been well characterized in terms of plasma kinetic and steady-state concentrations, mechanisms of anti-epileptic activity, and metabolism (Alvin and Bush 1977). However, the brain pharmacokinetics in relation to plasma drug levels were less well known, and the first human studies were done on samples of brain from neurosurgically treated epileptic patients. Most data on the distribution and kinetics of DPH in brain originated from animal studies (Stavchansky *et al.* 1978; Winstead *et al.* 1976). Now PET allows the determination of the pharmacokinetics of DPH in cerebral blood flow and brain tissue after intravenous injection of DPH labelled with carbon-11 (^{11}C, 20.4 min half-life).

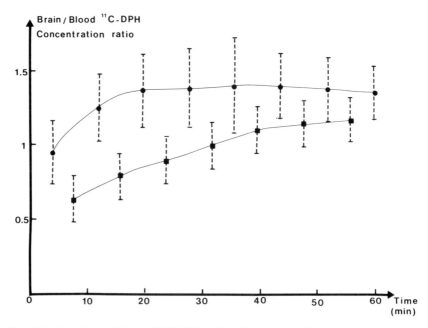

Fig. 5.1. Mean brain/blood [^{11}C]DPH radioactivity ratio with standard deviations plotted against time in ten human studies. ●, Grey matter; ■, white matter.

Fig. 5.1 shows the variations of brain/blood radioactivity ratio with time in ten patients with treatment-resistant epilepsy after an intravenous injection of 20 mCi of [^{11}C]DPH. It can be seen that in all the patients studied, white matter ^{11}C radioactivity levels were always lower than in grey matter. However, in the literature, in most animal and human studies, steady-state DPH concentration in white matter is equal or superior to that in grey matter (Stavchansky *et al.* 1978; Winstead *et al.* 1976), although these observations could not be reproduced by PET. This discrepancy can be explained by the fact that, in the PET experiments conducted in our laboratory, steady state could not be fully attained in white matter as a consequence of the fast physical decay of ^{11}C.

A basic assumption in PET studies is that the radioactivities in blood and brain really represent the labelled compound with a negligible amount coming from metabolites. In the case of labelled DPH this hypothesis is verified, for it has been shown that the radioactivity in blood and brain 1 h after injection is essentially unchanged DPH (Firemark *et al.* (1963).

Of the ten patients studied by PET, three were treated with therapeutic doses of DPH (i.e. 300 mg a day). From our results it is obvious that the brain uptake and kinetics of [¹¹C]DPH had not been affected by the current thera-peutic regime with DPH, in agreement with previous suggestions that the brain content of DPH is essentially not related to any specific binding sites (Goldber and Crandall 1978).

RECEPTOR-BINDING STUDIES

When the labelled drug is known to have an affinity for a particular receptor, PET gives the unique opportunity to visualize and to quantify *in vivo* the kinetics of the specific interaction of the radioligand with its receptor. In any receptor-binding study, the degree of specific radioactivity of the radioligand (i.e. radioactivity per unit mass) is of fundamental importance.

In PET studies, because of the relatively brief half-lives of the positron emitters used in the labelling process, specific radioactivities of the radio-ligands are theoretically extremely high. In fact they have to be high enough to allow the administration of a very small amount of tracer corresponding to a radioactivity that still can be accurately detected, after its distribution in the organism, by a positron camera.

As an example let us consider bromospiperone, a ligand labelled with the positron emitter bromine-76 (16.2 h half-life), and used for neuroleptic receptor studies. The theoretical specific radioactivity of the radiosotope is 200 Ci/μmol, but owing to various sources of contamination with stable bromine during the synthesis, the specific radioactivity of the radioligand is usually about one hundred times lower.

When 1 mCi of such a radioligand is injected intravenously in man, its concentration in the target organ (e.g. the brain) will be around 5×10^{-3} pmol/g of tissue for a total brain uptake of 1 per cent of the injected dose. In the basal ganglia, the dopamine receptor concentration is around 0.6 pmol/g of tissue (Bokobza *et al.* 1984); therefore only a small fraction (1/100) of these receptors will be saturated by the radioligand and in these conditions non-specific binding will be minimized.

Table 5.1 lists some of the molecules labelled with positron emitters used as ligands for *in vivo* visualization and quantification of brain functional systems containing specific binding sites. It is evident that when several radioligands are available for the same binding sites, the choice of the radionuclide will take into account the biological half-life of the phenomenon to be observed.

It is generally recognized that a binding site constitutes a receptor only if four conditions are simultaneously fulfilled, i.e. regional distribution, satur-ability, stereospecificity, and pharmacological or physiological effects. Demonstrations of these criteria in man or primate using PET technology and various labelled CNS-acting compounds will be described in the follow-ing paragraphs.

Regional distribution

The first example illustrating the characterization of a specific regional dis-tribution by PET is taken from a study on serotonin (5-hydroxytryptamine) receptors using ketanserin labelled with ¹¹C as a ligand (Baron *et al.* 1985).

TABLE 5.1. *Identification* in vivo *of receptor binding using positron emission tomography*

Receptor	References
1. Dopaminergic	
Chlorpromazine (^{11}C)	Comar *et al.* (1979)
	Mazière *et al.* (1975)
Bromospiperone (^{76}Br)	Mazière *et al.* (1984a)
Methylspiperone (^{11}C)	Wagner *et al.* (1983)
Fluorospiperone (^{18}F)	Welch *et al.* (1983)
Haloperidol (^{18}F)	Zanzonico *et al.* (1983)
Dopa (^{18}F)	Garnett *et al.* (1983)
2 Serotoninergic	
Ketanserin (^{11}C)	Laduron *et al.* (1982)
	Baron *et al.* (1985)
3. Opiate	
Etorphine (^{11}C)	Mazière *et al.* (1981a)
4. Benzodiazepine	
Diazepam (^{11}C)	Mazière *et al.* (1980)
Flunitrazepam (^{11}C)	Mazière *et al.* (1981b)
RO 15-1788 (^{11}C)	Hantraye *et al.* (1984)
PK 11-195 (^{11}C)	Camsonne *et al.* (1985)
5. β-Adrenergic	
Propranolol (^{11}C)	Berger *et al.* (1982)
Practolol (^{11}C)	Berger *et al.* (1983)
6. Muscarinic Cholinergic	
MQNB (^{11}C)	Mazière *et al.* (1981c)

Ketanserin, an antagonist of the serotonin (5-HT$_2$) receptors (Leysen *et al.* 1982), was labelled to high specific radioactivity (200 mCi/μmol) using [^{11}C]phosgene (Berridge *et al.* 1983). When 5-25 mCi of this labelled antagonist was injected intravenously into a man, the first image obtained 2 min after the tracer administration corresponded to a perfusion-like initial distribution, with a higher radioactivity in grey than in white matter. In control subjects, the early pattern of roughly equal radioactivity in the frontal cortex and the cerebellum progressively changed to a late appearance of higher radioactivity in the frontal cortex relative to cerebellum; this regional distribution probably reflected the higher density of 5-HT$_2$ receptors in the cortex than in the cerebellum.

The second example of regional localization of receptor sites by PET is taken from a study on benzodiazepine (BDZ) receptors, using as a ligand a BDZ antagonist, RO 15-1788 (RO 15) (Hantraye *et al.* 1984). For this study, RO 15 was labelled with ^{11}C([^{11}C]RO 15) with a high specific radioactivity (0.5-1.8 Ci/μmol) using a methylation process (Mazière *et al.*. 1980, 1984c).

The reasons for using a labelled BDZ antagonist such as [^{11}C]RO 15 for the '*in vivo*' study of brain BDZ receptors rather than a labelled BDZ agonist such as ^{11}Cflunitrazepam ([^{11}C]FLU) are as follows (Mazière *et al.* 1983) (1) the penetration of [^{11}C]RO 15 across the BBB is higher than that of [^{11}C]FLU; (2) the *in vivo* dissociation of the complex ligand–BDZ receptor is much slower with [^{11}C]RO 15 than with [^{11}C]FLU; (3) in contrast with [^{11}C]FLU, [^{11}C]RO 15, a ligand specific for central-type BDZ receptors, does not bind to peripheral-type BDZ receptors; (4) the absence of toxicity of the antagonist allows the administration of high doses of cold RO 15 in humans.

The studies were first performed in a baboon immobilized by injections of nortoxiferin (0.2–0.1 mg/kg), artificially ventilated, and placed supine in a painless position under a PET camera (Comar *et al.* 1981). Approximately 10 mCi (10 nmol) of [^{11}C]RO 15 was intravenously injected and measurements of the cerebral radioactivity were performed over 80 min.

As shown in Plate 5.1(a), the [^{11}C]RO 15 was not homogeneously distributed in brain. The brain radioactivity was mainly localized in the regions known to be rich in BDZ receptors: cerebellum (inferior part of the orbitomeatal (OM −0.5 slice), temporal and visual cortices (lateral and inferior area on the OM +1 slice), and frontal cortex (upper part of the OM +2.5 slice). This distribution remained constant during the entire course of the experiment. The brain kinetics of [^{11}C]RO 15 (Fig. 5.5, control curve) showed a high uptake of the drug in the brain, the maximum of which (5×10^{-4} of the injected dose) was reached within 10 min.

In man, after intravenous injection of 20 mCi of [^{11}C]RO 15, the radioactivity was mainly localized in cerebellar and temporal cortices (Plate 5.1b, left) and in occipital and frontal cortices (Plate 5.1b, right).

The criteria of specific binding site regional localization has also been demonstrated in human and primate for neuroleptic receptors using spiperone labelled with ^{11}C (Wagner *et al.* 1983), ^{18}F (Welch *et al.* 1983), bromine-77 (Owen *et al.* 1983), or bromine-76 (Mazière *et al.* 1983, 1984*a*).

In primate studies, when 2–5 mCi of bromospiperone labelled with bromine-76 ([^{76}Br]BSP) were intravenously injected into a baboon the sequential images obtained (Fig. 5.2) showed a progressive and relative concentration of the radioligand at the level of the basal ganglia. As seen in Fig. 5.3, the preferential accumulation of [^{76}Br]BSP was maximum 1.5 h after injection. At that time the striatum/cortex and striatum/cerebellum ratios were respectively 1.1 and 1.4. As the non-specifically bound ligand cleared from the cortex and the cerebellum these ratios increased with time, and 4.5 h post injection became equal to 1.5 and 2.2. It must be noticed that the spatial resolution of the positron camera compared to the size of the dopaminergic structures is such that partial volume effects produce an underestimation of these ratios.

The difference observed in the kinetics of elimination of [^{76}Br]BSP in cortex and striatum were probably due to the fact that in the striatum the radioligand bound nearly exclusively to dopamine receptors while in the cortex it bound also to 5-HT$_2$ receptors which are abundant in this structure.

In man, after the intravenous injection of 1–2 mCi of [^{76}Br]BSP the localization of the radioligand at the level of the striatum was particularly obvious

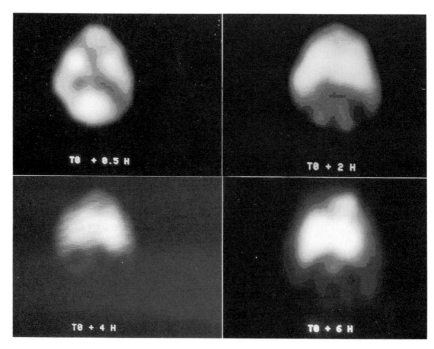

Fig. 5.2. PET images of baboon brain (OM + 1.5 cm) following intravenous injection of [^{76}Br]BSP (3 mCi, 1.1 Ci/μmol).

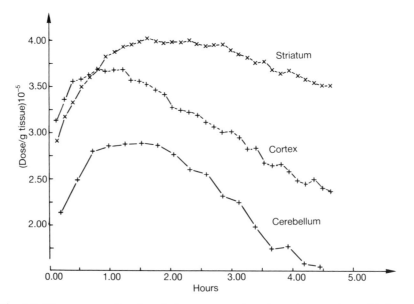

Fig. 5.3. Time course of radioactivity concentrations in various regions of baboon brain following intravenous injection of [^{76}Br]BSP (3.3 mCi, 1 Ci/μmol).

4 h post-injection (Fig. 5.4) when the non-specifically bound ligand had been eliminated. At that time the striatum to cerebellum ratio, which can be compared with the specific to non-specific binding ratio, was about 2.1.

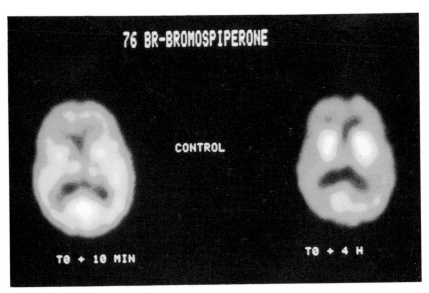

Fig. 5.4. PET images of one control study showing the changing pattern of [^{76}Br]BSP cerebral radioactivity with time. At the OM + 4.5 cm level the cortical radioactivity is initially higher than the striatal radioactivity but 4 h after injection the radioactive ligand is mostly concentrated in the striatum.

Saturability and stereospecificity

These criteria have been demonstrated in experiments at BDZ (Hantraye *et al.* 1984), 5-HT$_2$ (Baron *et al.* 1985) and (DA) receptor sites (Mazière *et al.* 1984*a*).

In BDZ-receptor-saturation studies in baboon, cold RO 15 co-injected with the radioligand induced a reduction in [^{11}C]RO 15 uptake by the brain in a dose-dependent mode (Fig. 5.5a). In displacement experiments, increasing doses of cold RO 15 injected 20 min after the radiotracer led to a dose-related decrease in brain radioactivity (Fig. 5.5b.). These displacements were also observed using a BDZ agonist such as lorazepam.

When using the D -isomer of an active BDZ, RO 11-6896, a high displacement was observed with a 0.5 mg/kg dose (Fig. 5.6); in contrast, no displacement was seen with the non-active isomer of the same BDZ (L -isomer, RO-11-6893) injected at the same very high dose.

To check the saturability and the stereospecificity of the binding of [^{76}Br]BSP to DA receptors, doses of cold antagonists (spiperone, (+)-butaclamol) were injected into a baboon 1.5 h before or after the administration

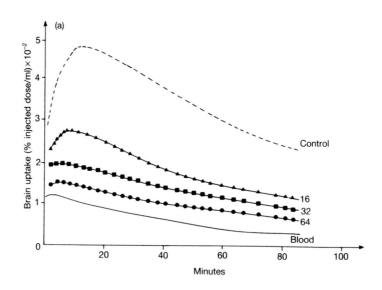

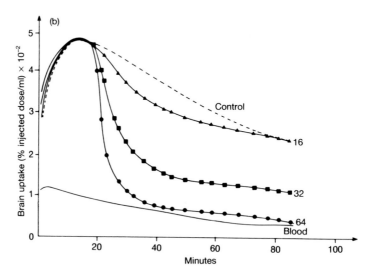

Fig. 5.5. Saturation (a) and displacement (b) experiments of [^{11}C]RO 15 cerebral binding. (a) [^{11}C]RO 15–1788 cerebral kinetics—change with co-injected increasing doses of RO 15–1788 (nmol/kg). (b) [^{11}C]RO 15–1788 cerebral kinetics—change with increasing doses of RO 15–1788 (nmol/kg) injected 20 min later.

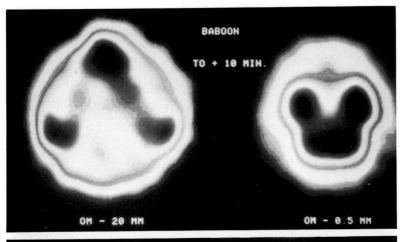

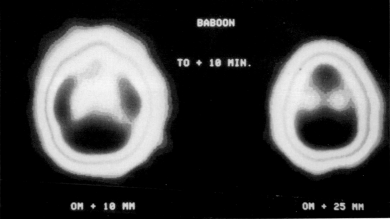

(a)

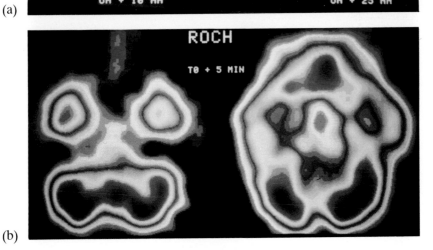

(b)

Plate 5.1. Brain distribution of the radioactivity 10 min after intravenous administration of [^{11}C]RO 15. (a) In a living baboon (10 mCi, four adjacent 12 mm brain slices); (b) in man (20 mCi), two 12 mm-thick slices including the cerebellar hemispheres (left) and the cerebral cortex (right).

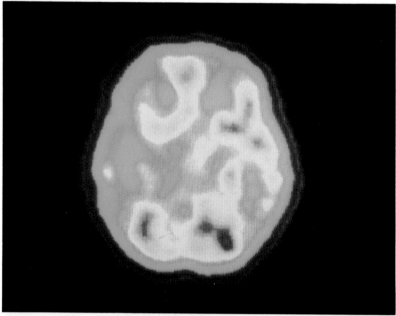

(a)

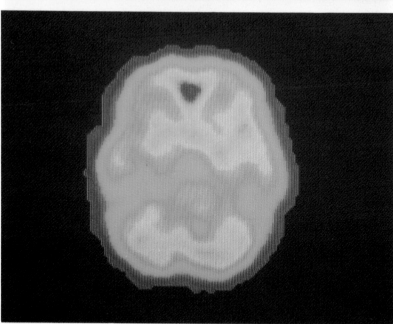

(b)

Plate 6.1. A PET scan showing changes following the administration of neuro-leptic medication. The patient was prescribed thioridazine for 1 month. Note the relative homogenization of contours after treatment. The patient was clinically improved when the second scan was taken.

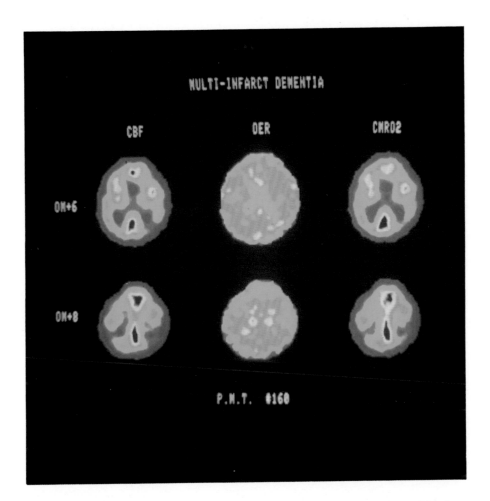

Plate 7.1. PET images showing CBF, CMRO₂, and OER in a patient with multi-infarct dementia. Note the multiple matched defects of flow and metabolism, such that OER is normal throughout the brain.

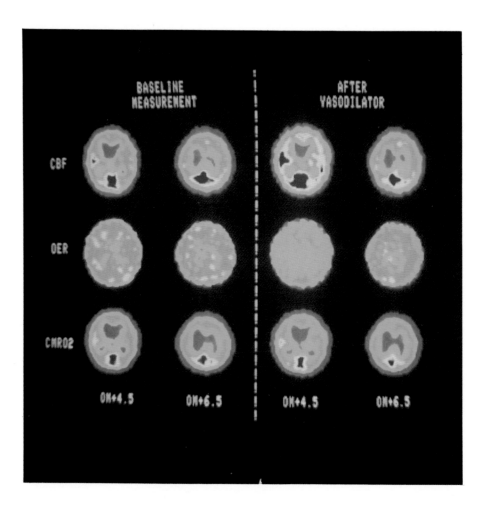

Plate 7.2. PET images in two tomographic planes before and after administration of the vasodilator drug. Note the transient rise of CBF and reciprocal fall of OER, evident only on the first tomographic slice (third column from left).

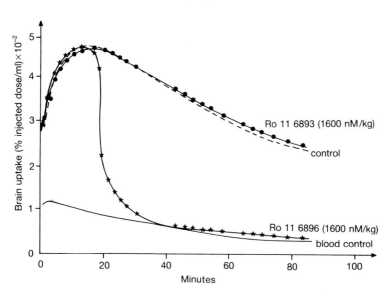

Fig. 5.6. Stereospecific displacement experiments in baboon after intravenous administration of a BDZ antagonist, [^{11}C]RO 15–1788 (10 mCi, 800–1000 mCi/μ mol). Cold loads of the two BDZ isomers RO 11–6893 and RO 11–6896 were injected 20 min after the radioligand. Brain radioactivity was registered by PET at the level OM + 1 cm.

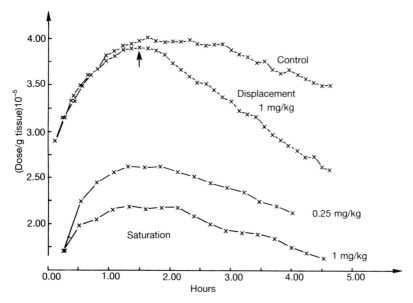

Fig. 5.7. Time course of radioactivity concentrations in the striatum of baboon following intravenous injections of [^{76}Br]BSP (3–4 mCi). Effects of unlabelled spiperone administered 1.5 h before or following (added at arrow) the radioligand injection.

of the radioligand. The influence of these cold loads of spiperone on the brain kinetics of [^{76}Br]BSP is illustrated in Fig. 5.7. In the striatal region, 1 mg/kg of spiperone administered once the ligand concentration reached a plateau displaced the binding of the radioactive tracer, while progressive cold loads of the same antagonist administered 1.5 h before the radioligand gradually saturated the DA receptors leading to a diminution of the binding of [^{76}Br]BSP in the striatum. In the same way this specifically bound radioactivity was displaced by the active isomer of butaclamol at a dose of 1 mg/kg.

Such competitive displacement in humans is always difficult to perform because of the pharmacological effects of the cold drugs which have to be injected in therapeutic doses to fully saturate the binding sites studied. Nevertheless for neurotransmitter receptors, the *in vivo* saturability of the binding sites can be demonstrated in patients treated with high doses of neuroleptics. For example in the previous study on 5-HT$_2$ receptors with [^{11}C]ketanserin, four treated schizophrenics were studied 2 h after intramuscular injection of cold chlorpromazine (CPZ) in therapeutic doses (70 mg). PET measurements show a lower uptake and faster kinetics of elimination of the radioligand in the frontal cortex of these pretreated patients than in controls. These significant differences can be explained by an almost full occupation of the 5-HT$_2$ receptors by the large doses of CPZ administered to the patients.

Another example comes from our work on brain neuroleptic receptors. When the ligand [^{76}Br]BSP was injected into schizophrenics pretreated with doses of haloperidol (10 mg, intramuscularly) high enough to saturate the neuroleptic-binding sites in the brain, it was no longer possible to visualize the dopamine-binding sites in the basal ganglia using PET (the striatum to cerebellum radioactivity ratio 4 h after the administration of the tracer was only 1.3).

Pharmacological effects

This last criterion allows discrimination between acceptors and receptors for there is no receptor that has no physiological or pharmacological response.

Correlation between pharmacological activity and receptor occupancy, which is the decisive criterion of specificity, has been demonstrated directly and indirectly in baboons for the BDZ receptors: (1) indirectly—a correlation was found between the amount of [^{11}C]RO 15 radioactivity displaced in the cerebellum by increasing doses of cold RO 15 and the increasing quantity of pentamethylenetetrazol necessary to induce, in the same animal, generalized seizures (Mazière *et al.* 1984*a*) (2) directly—when the brain [^{11}C]RO 15 radioactivity was displaced by a convulsant drug known to act at the level of BDZ receptors such as methyl-β-carbolinecarboxylate (βCCM), the intensity of the displacement observed by PET was correlated with an increase in brain electrical activity (EEG) (Fig. 5.8); the importance of the two phenomena was directly related to the dose of cold βCCM administered intravenously.

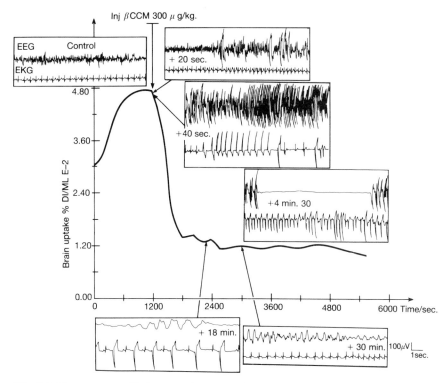

Fig. 5.8. Time course of baboon brain radioactivity concentrations following intravenous administration of [^{11}C]RO 15 (10 mCi, 800 mCi/μmol); effects of cold βCCM (300μg/kg) injected intravenously 20 min after the radioligand on brain radioactivity and on brain electrical activity (EEG).

CONCLUSIONS

The first example described studies with [^{11}C]DPH and demonstrated the ability of PET to provide tissue pharmacokinetics non-invasively in humans.

In other examples related to receptor-binding studies, the experimental results convincingly demonstrate that the kinetics are directly related to specific binding of ligands to brain receptors. Displacement or competition experiments allow differentiation of specific from non-specific components.

Nevertheless as equilibrium conditions are never achieved *in vivo*, equations used *in vitro* to quantify the binding parameters are not appropriate for the treatment of PET values. So, to study quantitatively the kinetics of specific binding *in vivo*, a mathematical model has been recently derived from experimental results on muscarinic heart receptor binding (Syrota *et al.* 1984). This model, which tries to explain the somewhat conflicting findings of *in vitro* and *in vivo* experiments, explains the receptor-occupancy-dependent dissociation rate observed *in vivo* by the probability that the ligand will rebind to receptors, owing to the existence of a boundary layer close to the cell membranes where the receptors are located.

Using this model it should be possible to evaluate through PET studies and sequential results the values of the kinetic parameters which characterize any specific binding of ligands to receptors.

ACKNOWLEDGEMENTS

The authors wish to thank the staff of the Service Hospitalier Frédéric Joliot for their collaboration and N. De Blecker for her help in preparing the manuscript. This work was partly supported by CNRS grant (ATP no. 031927).

REFERENCES

Alvin, J. D. and Bush, M. T. (1977). Diphenylhydantoins and other hydantoins. In *Anticonvulsants* (ed. J. A. Vida), 116 pp. Academic Press, New York.

Baron, J. C., Roeda, D., Munari, C., Crouzel, C., Chodkiewicz, J. P., and Comar, D. (1983*a*). Brain regional pharmacokinetics of ^{11}C-labeled diphenylhydantoin: positron emission tomography in humans. *Neurology* **33**, 580–5.

—— Comar, D., Zarifian, E., Crouzel, C., Mestelan, G., Loo, H., and Agid, Y. (1983*b*). An *in vivo* study of the dopaminergic receptors in the brain of man using ^{11}C-pimozide and positron emission tomography. In *Functional radionuclide imaging of the brain* (ed. P. L. Magistretti), pp. 337–45. Raven Press, New York.

—— Samson, Y., Crouzel, C., Berridge, M., Chretien, L., Denicker, P., Comar, D., and Agid, Y. (1985). Pharmacologic studies in man with PET: an investigation using ^{11}C-labeled ketanserin, a 5HT$_2$ receptor antagonist. In *Measurement of cerebral blood flow and cerebral metabolism in man.* Springer-Verlag, Berlin (in press).

Berger, G., Prenant, C., Sastre, J., Syrota, A., and Comar, D. (1983). Synthesis of a β-blocker for heart visualization: (^{11}C) practolol. *Int. J. Appl. Radiat. Isot.* **34 (11)**, 1556.

—— Mazière, M., Prenant, C., Sastre, J., Syrota, A., and Comar, D. (1982). Synthesis of ^{11}C-propanolol. *J. Radioanal. Chem.* **74**, 301–6.

Berridge, M., Comar, D., Crouzel, C., and Baron, J. C. (1983). ^{11}C-labelled ketanserin, a selective serotonin S$_2$ antagonist. *J. Label. Comp. Radiopharm.* **20**, 73–8.

Bokobza, B., Ruberg, M., Scatton, B., Javoy-Agid, F., and Agid, Y. (1984). (^{3}H) spiperone binding, dopamine and HVA concentrations in Parkinson's disease and supranuclear palsy. *Europ. J. Pharmacol.* **99**, 167–75.

Camsonne, R., Crouzel, C., Comar, D., Mazière, M., Prenant, C., Sastre, J., Moulijn, M. A. and Syrota, A. (1985). Synthesis of *N*-(^{11}C) methyl *N*(methyl-1 propyl) (chloro-2 phenyl)-1-isoquinoleine carboxamide-3 (PK 11195): a new ligand for peripheral benzodiazepine receptors. *J. Label. Comp. Radiopharm.* (in press).

Comar, D. and Mazière, M. (1982). An approach for the study of specific binding *in vivo*, using positron computed tomography. In *Radionuclide imaging*, pp. 263–88. Pergamon Press, France.

—— —— Cepeda, C., Godot, J. M., Menini, C., and Naquet, R. (1981). The kinetics and displacement of (^{11}C)flunitrazepam in the brain of the living baboon. *Europ. J. Pharmacol.* **75**, 21–6.

—— Zarifian, E., Verhas, M., (1979). Brain distribution and kinetics of ^{11}C-chlorpromazine in schizophrenics: positron emission tomography studies. *Psychiat. Res.* **1**, 23–9.

Firemark, H., Barlow, C. F., and Roth, L. J. (1963). The entry, accumulation and binding of diphehylhydantoin-2-C^{14} in brain studies on adult, immature and hypercapnic cats. *Int. J. Neuropharmacol.* **2**, 25–38.

Garnett, E. S., Firnau, G., and Nahmias, C. (1983). Dopamine visualized in the basal ganglia of living man. *Nature, Lond.* **305**, 137.

Goldber, M. A. and Crandall, P. H. (1978). Human brain binding of phenytoin. *Neurology* **28**, 881–5.

Hantraye, P., Kaijima, M., Prenant, C., Guibert, B., Sastre, J., Crouzel, M., Naquet, R., Comar, D., and Mazière, M. (1984). Central type benzodiazepine binding sites: a positron emission tomography study in the baboon's brain. *Neurosci. Lett.* **48**, 115–20.

Laduron, P. M., Janssen, P. F. M., and Leysen, J. E. (1982). *Europ. J. Pharmacol.* **81**, 43–8.

Leysen, J. E., Niemegeers, C. J. E., Van Nueten, J. M., and Laduron, P. M. (1982). ^{3}H-ketanserin (R 41 468), a selective ligand for serotonin 2, receptor binding sites. Binding properties, brain distribution and functional role. *Molec. Pharmacol.* **21**, 301–4.

Mazière, B., Loc'h, C., Hantraye, P., Guillon, R., Duquesnoy, N., Soussaline, F., Naquet, R., Comar, D., and Mazière, M. (1984*a*). ^{76}Br-bromospiroperidol: a new tool for quantitative *in-vivo* imaging of neuroleptic receptors. *Life Sci.* **35**. 1349–56.

—— Berger, G., and Comar, D. (1982). ^{11}C-radiopharmaceuticals for brain receptors studies in conjunction with positron emission tomography. In *Application of nuclear and radiochemistry* (eds R. M. Lambrecht and N. Morcos), pp. 251–70. Pergamon Press, New York.

—— Sainte-Laudy, J. L., Crouzel, M., and Comar, D. (1975). Synthesis and distribution kinetics of ^{11}C chlorpromazine in animals. In *Radiopharmaceuticals* (ed. G. Subramian), pp. 189–95, Society of Nuclear Medicine.

—— Godot, J. M., Berger, G., Prenant, C., and Comar, D. (1980). High specific activity carbon-11 labelling of benzodiazepines: diazepam and flunitrazepam. *J. Radioanal. Chem.* **56**, 229–35.

—— —— —— and —— (1981*a*). ^{11}C-labelled etorphine for *in vivo* studies of opiate receptors in brain. *J. Radioanal. Chem.* **62**, 279–84.

—— Hantraye, P., Prenant, C., Sastre, J., and Comar, D. (1984c). RO 15 1788-^{11}C: a specific radioligand for "*in vivo*" central benzodiazepine receptor study by positron emission tomography. *Int. J. Appl. Radiat. Isotop.* **35**, 973–6.

—— Comar, D., Godot, J. M., Collard, P., Cepeda, C., and Naquet, R. (1981*c*). *In vivo* characterization of myocardium muscarinic receptors by positron emission tomography. *Life Sci.* **29**, 2391–7.

—— Godot, J. M., Berger, G., Baron, J. C., Comar, D., Cepeda, C., Menini, C., and Naquet, R. (1981*b*). Positron tomography a new method for *in vivo* brain studies of benzodiazepine in animal and in man. In *GABA and benzodiazepine receptors* (ed. E. Costa). Raven Press, New York.

—— Hantraye, P., Guibert, B., Kaijima, M., Prenant, C., Sastre, J., Crouzel, M., Naquet, R., and Comar, D. (1984*b*). RO 15 1788-^{11}C: a specific radioligand for an "*in vivo*" study of central benzodiazepine receptors, by positron emission tomography. *Clin. Neuropharmacol.* **7**, *Suppl.* **1**, 662–3.

—— Prenant, C., Sastre, J., Crouzel, M., Comar, D., Hantraye, P., Kaïjima, M., Guibert, B., and Naquet, R. (1983). ^{11}C-RO 15-1788 et ^{11}C-flunitrazepam, deux coordinat-spour l'étude par tomographie par positons des sites de liaison des benzodiazé-pines. *C. R. Acad. Sci. (Paris) Sér. III* **296**, 871–6.

Owen, F., Poulter, M., Mashal, R. D., Crow, T. J., Veall, N., and Zanelli, G. D. (1983). ^{77}Br-p-spiperone: a ligand for *in-vivo* labelling of dopamine receptors. *Life Sci.* **33**, 765–8.

Phelps, M. E. (1977). Emission computed tomography. *Semin. Nucl. Med.* **7**, 337–65.

Ramsay, R. E. (1983). Valproate brain tissue kinetics determined by PET. *Neurology* **33**, *Suppl.* **2**, 147.

Stavchansky, S. A., Tilbury, R. S. McDonald, J. M. Ting, C. T., and Kostenbauder, H. B. *In vivo* distribution of carbon-11 phenytoin and its major metabolite and their use in scintigraphic imaging. *J. Nucl. Med.* **19**, 936–41.

Syrota, A., Paillotin, G., Davy, J. M., Aumont, M. C. (1984). Kinetics of *in vivo* binding of antagonist to muscarinic cholinergic receptor in the human heart studied by positron emission tomography. *Life Sci.* **35**, 937–45.

Ter-Pogossian, M. M., Phelps, M. E., Hoffmann, E. J., and Mullani, N. A. (1975). A positron-emission transaxial tomograph for nuclear imaging (PETT). *Radiology* **114**, 89–98.

Wagner, Jr. H. N., Burns, H. D., Dannals, R. F., Wong, D. F., Langstrom, B., Duelfer, T., Frost, J. J., Ravert, H. T., Links, J. M., Rosenbloom, S. B., Lukas, S. E., Kramer, A. F., and Kuhar, M. J. (1983). Imaging dopamine receptors in the human brain by positron tomography. *Science* **221**, 1264–6.

Welch, M. J., Kilbourn, M. R., Mathias, C. J., Mintun, M. A., and Raichle, M. E. (1983). *Life Sci.* **33**, 1687–93.

Winstead, M. B., Parr, S. J., and Royal, M. J. (1976). Relationship of molecular structure to *in vivo* scintigraphic distribution patterns of carbon-11 labeled compounds-3-^{11}C) hydantoins. *J. Med. Chem.* **19**, 279–86.

Yamamoto, Y. L., Diksic, M., Sako, K., Arita, N., Feindel, W., and Thompson, C. J. (1983). Pharmacokinetic and metabolic studies in human malignant glioma. In *Functional radionuclide imaging of the brain* (ed. P. L. Magistretti), pp. 327–35. Raven Press, New York.

Zanzonico, P. B., Bigler, R. E., and Schmall, B. (1983). Neuroleptic binding sites: specific labeling in mice with (^{18}F)-haloperidol a potential tracer for positron-emission tomogrpahy. *J. Nucl. Med.* **24**, 408–16.

6

Positron emission tomography scanning in epilepsy with special reference to psychoses

MICHAEL R. TRIMBLE

INTRODUCTION

The introduction of PET scanning in the last few years, the methodology of which is described in other chapters in this monograph, has led important investigations regarding brain function in epilepsy to be carried out. Much of the pioneering work in this field has been undertaken by Engel and colleagues (Engel *et al.* 1982*a*) and most of the studies have used the 18-fluorodeoxy-glucose method. Both ictal and interictal studies have been undertaken, and attempts have been made to correlate changes noted on PET scanning with EEG and underlying neuropathological variables. Other groups have used oxygen-15-labelled H_2O and O_2 (Bernard *et al.* 1983; Depresseux *et al.* 1983), and the accumulated data can be compared with other studies using dynamic imaging, including single-photon-emission-computed tomography (SPECT), and cerebral blood flow studies with Xenon-133 (Lavy *et al.* 1976; Sanabria *et al.* 1983). It seems clear from these studies that imaging techniques such as PET scanning are providing information about brain function in epilepsy hitherto unsuspected, and that these data compliment and extend information gleaned from other techniques, for example electro-encephalography or CT scanning.

Early observations, for example during craniotomies in patients with epilepsy undergoing cerebral surgery, indicated that an increase in blood flow was seen in association with epileptic discharges (Penfield and Jasper 1954), and with the introduction of the nitrous oxide method of Kety and Schmidt (1948), estimation of cerebral blood flow in the total human brain during epileptic seizures became possible. Initial studies confirmed an increase in both cerebral blood flow (CBF) and the cerebral metabolic rate of oxygen use ($CMRO_2$) during epileptic seizures and the introduction of regional CBF (rCBF) analysis confirmed a focal region of increase correlating to the site of the abnormal EEG discharges (Ingvar 1975).

In contrast to these data during the ictus, interictal studies provided less clear information. Thus, the interictal CBF in epilepsy was reported as normal (Grant *et al.* 1947), increased (Hougaard and Oikawa 1975), and decreased (Lavy *et al.* 1976). Some of the problems encountered with rCBF studies, including the fact that only lateral parts of the cortex are perceived, have been overcome with PET scanning, evaluating brain function in three dimensions, and providing quantitative regional data during different clinical states.

PET STUDIES

Engel *et al.* (1982*a*) reported data on the interictal cerebral glucose metabolism in 50 patients with partial epilepsy under evaluation for possible surgical resection of their epileptogenic lesions. In their studies, PET scanning is performed with concurrent EEG recording either from scalp electrodes or with stereotaxically implanted depth electrodes. Seventy per cent of their scans revealed one or more areas of abnormal hypometabolism, which in many was localized to the temporal cortex. Only one patient showed a possible increase in interictal metabolism and this was noted within a hypometabolic zone. Using the spike frequency detected from direct counting of EEG records, they were unable to reveal any correlation between electroencephalographic data and the relative amount of hypometabolism in the abnormal brain areas. Generally, however, when all available EEG recordings were combined to arrive at an electrophysiological localization of the epileptogenic focus, good agreement was seen with the location of the hypometabolic areas detected with PET scanning. Complete disagreement was noted in only 6 per cent of patients, but only in one case was the PET scan suspected of producing falsely localized results. False negatives, that is patients who went on to have surgery, thus confirming a pathological underpinning for the seizures, but who on examination had normal PET scans, were seen in only two cases, which were attributable to technically inadequate scans.

In a further study (Engel *et al.* 1982*b*) the pathological findings underlying focal temporal hypometabolism were studied in 25 patients who underwent resection. Pathological lesions were found in 19 removed temporal lobes, in 15 the pathology was mesial temporal sclerosis involving the hippocampus, the dentate gyrus, and the subiculum. All 19 patients showed a zone of hypometabolism on their scans in the temporal lobe operated on prior to operation, and the most interesting finding was that the zones of hypometabolism noted with PET scanning were much larger in most cases than the pathological lesions demonstrated by conventional histological methods. Typically the entire temporal lobe on the side of the focus was found to be hypometabolic and artifactual causes for this have been ruled out. Engel *et al.* (1984*a, b*) have argued that this extensive hypometabolism thus represents an anatomical or functional property of the epileptogenic focus itself, either based on structural abnormalities unidentified by routine pathological examination or on 'functional suppression of glucose utilization due either to inhibition or inactivation of relatively healthy neuronal elements or else to variants in vascular profusion'.

The reversibility of these lesions has been demonstrated in two ways. First, some patients have been examined in the ictal and interictal states, and ictal activation of zones of interictal hypometabolism have been demonstrated (Mazziotta and Engel 1984). Secondly, Gur *et al.* (1982) have carried out positron emission tomography in two cases of the Lennox–Gastaut syndrome who underwent corpus callosum section for their seizures. Both patients demonstrated preoperative areas of hypometabolism, which persisted after the operation in one of the patients who obtained no benefit from the surgery. In the other, however, who clinically improved, the hypometabolism resolved.

Theodore *et al.* (1983) have also reported interictal studies in epilepsy in a series of patients using the fluorodeoxyglucose technique, and they generally confirm the findings of Engel and colleagues. In particular they find no correlation between the observed hypometabolism and either seizure frequency, duration of the seizure disorder, the presence of multiple seizure types or occurrence of secondary generalized seizures.

OXYGEN STUDIES

In collaboration with the Hammersmith Hospital, London, my colleagues and I have reported an interictal study of partial epilepsy using positron emission tomography and oxygen-15 (Bernardi *et al.* 1983). In this study, ten patients with complex partial seizures, selected because they demonstrated on clinical examination, or on electroencephalography, evidence of a temporal lobe focus, were scanned and their data compared with age-matched healthy controls with no known neurological disease. In contrast to the fluorodeoxyglucose method, the oxygen technique allows for evaluation of rCBF, $rCMRO_2$, and the relationship between blood flow and oxygen utilzation, namely the rOER (see Chapter 2). Using this method we were able to confirm the findings of Engel and colleagues of an extensive area of hypometabolism in patients with complex partial seizures deriving from the temporal lobe, in our studies the hypometabolism being associated with low cerebral blood flow and being seen maximally on the side of the focus in regions of interest from the frontal lobe, the posterior temporal lobe, and the basal ganglia (see Fig. 6.1). Further, by comparison with expected values from normal controls, the contralateral temporal cortex also had diminished values for rCBF and $rCMRO_2$ (see Fig. 6.2) although this was less extensive than in the ipsilateral hemisphere. The cerebellum was also examined and the rCBF and the $rCMRO_2$ was significantly decreased in the epileptic patients in both hemispheres. These data confirmed and extended therefore the findings from Engel *et al.* (1982*a,b*) notably by demonstrating: that the abnormalities detected with the fluorodeoxyglucose technique were replicable with oxygen studies; that the areas of hypometabolism were extensively distributed beyond the supposed area of pathological abnormality in the temporal lobe patients with complex partial seizures, even in a group that were not awaiting surgery and who therefore had a less-severe seizure disorder; that the functional changes extend to the basal ganglia and frontal cortices in addition to the temporal cortex; that the cerebellum may be

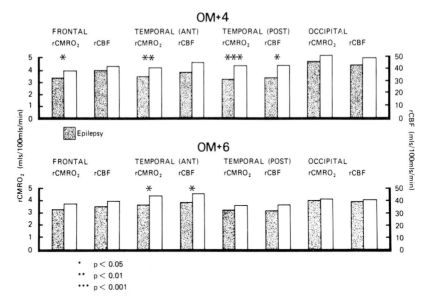

Fig. 6.1. This shows the rCBF and rCMRO$_2$ in the ipsilateral hemisphere on two slices OM+4 and OM+6. Patients had mainly unilateral abnormalities on surface electroencephalograms, and it demonstrates widespread hypometabolism and low blood flow in the epileptic patients compared with controls. Speckled, epilepsy; plain, control.

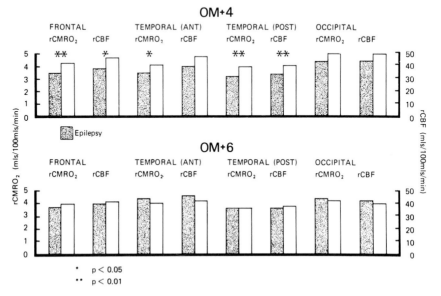

Fig. 6.2. Showing the rCBF and rCMRO$_2$ in the contralateral hemisphere in the same patients as Fig. 1. Again significant differences are seen, although less widespread in the epileptic patients.

involved more fundamentally in the seizure disorder than otherwise suspected; and that contralateral changes are also noted, although being less severe than on the side of the focus.

Interestingly, in the temporal cortex on the side of the focus a significant increase in the rOER was reported. The relevance of this was not clear, but it may reflect a diminished reserve of oxygen supply to this area of brain suggesting an increased vulnerability of neurons in this region to decreased perfusion or oxygenation of the arterial blood during subsequent seizures.

Yamamoto and colleague (1984) have published data on 14 patients using both radioactively labelled glucose and oxygen, and note in general a similarity in findings using the two techniques, and again confirm zones of hypometabolism interictally in patients with partial seizures.

In contrast to these studies on partial epilepsy, there are very few investigators who have examined the interictal state of patients with generalized epilepsy. In our own studies, three patients with primary generalized epilepsy and a history of tonic/clonic seizures have been examined in the interictal state, the same methodology being employed as that described for the other studies (see Bernardi *et al.* 1983). The results from the temporal cortex of these three patients and the corresponding values for age-matched controls are shown in Table 6.1. It can be seen that the interictal values obtained are within the normal range. These preliminary data would suggest that the interictal hypometabolism, so clearly described for partial-seizure patients, may not be apparent in all forms of epilepsy, and that patients with generalized epilepsy may show relatively few interictal disturbances. This has particular significance for the links between epilepsy and psychiatry, in the sense that the history of this association has revolved mainly around temporal lobe epilepsy and patients with partial seizures (Trimble 1981). This is further considered below in the discussion of epileptic psychosis.

TABLE 6.1. *A comparison of the means for rCBF, rCMRO$_2$, and rOER (ml 100 ml^{-1} min^{-1}) for the temporal cortex; generalized (G) vs complex partial seizures (TL). (Interictal scans).*

	rCBF		rCMRO$_2$		rOER	
	G	TL	G	TL	G	TL
(Mean)	($n=3$)	($n=5$)	($n=3$)	($n=5$)	($n=3$)	($n=5$)
Frontal	4.0	3.2	43.0	35.9	0.45	0.52
Temporal (ant)	5.0	3.7	57.0	41.8	0.48	0.53
Temporal (post)	4.8	3.3	46.4	35.8	0.52	0.54
Occipital	4.2	3.8	40.7	41.1	0.47	0.57
Basal Ganglia	5.2	3.7	55.6	44.7	0.48	0.47

ICTAL STUDIES

In contrast to the interictal hypometabolism described with partial seizures, several patients have been studied during the ictal state (Mazziotta and Engel 1984). All have been with glucose, and the technical limitations of the measurements obtained with high rates of glucose metabolism which obtained during seizures are less than certain. Generally, scans obtained during partial seizures show hypermetabolic areas which correspond to the areas of hypometabolism noted interictally. Interestingly Engel *et al.* (1983) report a relative reduction in metabolic activity at areas distant from the ictal hypermetabolism, the meaning of which is not entirely clear. Absence seizures and iatrogenically induced seizures with ECT have also been studiedied using the deoxyglucose technique (Mazziotta and Engel 1984). During a generalized absence episode diffuse increases in the uptake of glucose are seen, the degree of hypermetabolism not correlating with the frequency or duration of the clinical episodes. Four patients were studied following ECT, the scan being obtained by injecting the fluorodeoxyglucose at the time of the bilateral electroshock. The cerebral metabolic rate is generally increased over expected values with ECT, although if deoxyglucose is given post-ictally diffuse hypometabolism is noted, particularly in cortical structures. These data with positron emission tomography in patients undergoing ECT compliment those of Silfverskiöld *et al.* (1984), who have demonstrated, using xenon-133 that the rCBF decreases following ECT, the results being less pronounced and asymmetrical if unilateral electrode placement is used.

ANTI–CONVULSANT DRUGS

There are few studies of the effects of anti-convulsant drugs on blood flow and metabolism in patients. Theodore *et al.* (1983) attempted to relate changes in the background frequency of the EEG to seizure frequency, medication, and frontal hypometabolism on PET scans. However, medication and clinical manifestations were reported to be similar in patients with or without frontal hypometabolism, and thus they did not relate their findings to an effect of medication. Bernardi *et al.* (1983) commented that six of their ten patients with partial seizures were on phenytoin, one was on no therapy, and two were on carbamazepine monotherapy. The mean values of the $CMRO_2$ for the patients on carbamazepine were higher than the group mean. Baron *et al.* (1983) synthesized [^{11}C]phenytoin and gave it to epileptic patients in an attempt to evaluate further phenytoin pharmacokinetics within the epileptic focus. The uptake of the radioactive phenytoin was higher in grey matter than white matter, presumably reflecting the higher perfusion rate of the former, and was within previously reported ranges for normal brain areas. Thus although the radioactive phenytoin was noted to be present in the focus, it was ineffective in the sense that these patients were still continuing to have persistant seizures. Clearly further studies of the effects of anti-convulsants on rCBF and metabolism in man are required, not only with a view to understanding further how these compounds act upon a seizure focus, but also so that the abnormal findings from the ictal and interictal studies of epileptic patients can be better evaluated. Thus, with few exceptions, all of the patients in the literature where PET scanning has been used in epilepsy have been medicated. The fact that patients with generalized seizures do not appear to show the demonstrated areas of focal hypometabolism seen in focal epilepsy, and the correlation of the maximum areas of hypometabolism interictally in this group with EEG indications of where the focus might be suggest that the administration of anti-convulsant drugs is not however the major factor determining these abnormalities.

EPILEPTIC PSYCHOSES

The relationship between epilepsy and psychoses has been much debated for a long time. Although descriptions are available from the last century, most interest in this subject has recurred since the 1950s with the writings of authors such as Hill (1953), Pond (1957), and Slater and Beard (1963). These authors confirm that certain forms of psychoses, particularly those with a schizophreniform presentation, occur in epileptic patients, and are more frequently seen in patients with temporal lobe abnormalities. Although much further work needs to be done, there is growing evidence that a schizophreniform psychosis of epilepsy is associated with intractable seizures that start in childhood, with a medial as opposed to lateral temporal lobe focus, and with a focus of abnormality lateralized to the dominant hemisphere. (For review see Trimble 1984.) In order to evaluate cerebral metabolic changes in patients with epileptic psychosis, we have carried out PET scanning with ^{15}O and compared the data to an age-matched non-psychotic epileptic group who also had complex partial seizures. Further, we have evaluated a third group of patients, who were also psychotic and had epilepsy, but were being treated with neuroleptic medication in addition to their anti-convulsant drugs.

Materials and methods

The three groups consisted of the following patients. Group one consisted of psychotic epileptic patients ($n = 6$) all with complex partial seizures, none of whom were being treated with neuroleptic medication. The second group ($n = 6$) was also psychotic, but was receiving neuroleptic medication, while the third group ($n = 5$) comprised age-matched non-psychotic epileptic patients with temporal lobe epilepsy. In all patients except one the psychosis was rated using the Present State Examination PSE of Wing (Wing *et al.* 1974) and the scans were taken interictally. Three patients were scanned on two occasions, once on a neuroleptic drug, and once drug-free.

The scan procedure has been described elsewhere (Frackowiak *et al.* 1980) and will not be outlined here. In the majority of patients and the controls, scanning was carried out at OM (orbito-meatal line) +2, +4, +6, and +8 cm. All were corrected for attenuation by the corresponding transmission scans, and tracer equations which relate steady-state measurements to tissue blood flow and oxygen extraction ratios were used to calculate absolute quantative values of rCBF, rOER, adn rCMRO$_2$.

Following a printout from the computer, quantitative data representing 2.5 cm^{2}regions of interest were chosen and analysed corresponding to the frontal and occipital regions on slices at OM+4 and OM+6 respectively. Three areas were measured from the temporal cortex, each of 1.5 cm^2 in a continuous strip on slice OM+4. Additional areas examined included a 'fronto-temporal bridge' (representing an island of cortical tissue between the frontal and temporal areas on slice OM+4) and the basal ganglia. The latter was estimated using a 41 pixel Region Of Interest directly from the visual display unit on which scans were projected. Statistical analysis of the data was by Student's *t* test, one way ANOVA, and the post hoc means test.

TABLE 6.2. *Some parameters of the groups investigated.*

	Mean age (years)	Mean IQ	Mean seizures/ month
Epileptic, non psychotic	34.0	98	9.2*
Epileptic, psychotic	38.2	97	3.9
Epileptic, psychotic; on neuroleptics	42.3	96	1.4

* One patient had 30.

The mean ages, IQs, and seizure frequencies of the groups are shown in Table 6.2. No statistical differences were noted between them. The PSE ratings were nuclear schizophrenia (NS) for four of the untreated group (a fifth patient, not given the PSE also had nuclear schizophrenia) and two of the treated group. The neuroleptic-drug-free psychotic patients had no neuroleptic medication for varying intervals. In one patient this was 9 days, in the second 24 days, in two others over 7 months and two patients had never received any such treatment before. When the cortical areas for the frontal, temporal, and occipital areas were examined, all three of these epileptic samples showed consistently lower values for rCBF and rCMRO$_2$, compared with a non-epileptic volunteer population, maximal differences being noted in the more posterior temporal areas. When the psychotic, non-neuroleptic treated, and the non-psychotic epileptic control groups were compared the psychotic patients had lower rCMRO$_2$, higher rCBF, and lower rOER values, the differences appearing in a constant pattern over the majority of areas. Significantly lower rOERs were recorded in the following regions on both sides: frontal, temporal, fronto-temporal bridge, basal ganglia, and limbic strip. When laterality differences were examined it was noted that the non-neuroleptically treated psychotic group showed lower values for the rCBF and rCMRO$_2$ on the left side across the entire temporal cortex, findings not seen in the non-psychotic control group (see Fig. 6.3 and Table 6.3).

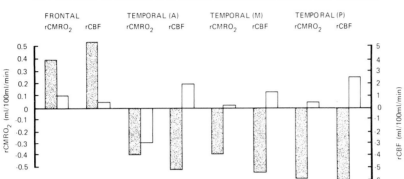

Fig. 6.3. Absolute differences in the rCMRO$_2$ and rCBF in patients who are psychotic and those who are non-psychotic, both groups having epilepsy. There is significant down-regulation of activity in the temporal regions, maximal posteriorly, in the psychotic group. Speckled, psychotic; plain, non-psychotic.

TABLE 6.3. *Values of left–right side comparing the epileptic non-psychotic to the epileptic psychotic group.*

		EP	Control	Significance
Frontal	CMRO$_2$	+0.4	+0.1	0.10
	CBF	+5.4	+0.3	0.04
	OER	0	0	
Temporal (A)	CMRO$_2$	−0.4	−0.3	
	CBF	−5.2	−1.9	
	OER	−0.01	−0.05	0.02
Temporal (M)	CMRO$_2$	0.6	0	0.05
	CBF	−5.7	−1.1	
	OER	−0.01	−0.03	
Temporal (P)	CMRO$_2$	−0.6	0	0.06
	CBF	−7.2	+2.6	0.06
	OER	−0.01	−0.04	
FTCB	CMRO$_2$	−0.3	0	
	CBF	−3.5	+2.4	0.10
	OER	−0.01	−0.02	
Occipital	CMRO$_2$	−0.3	−0.4	
	CBF	−4.7	−3.0	
	OER	0	0	
Basal ganglia	CMRO$_2$	−0.2	−0.0	
	CBF	−2.5	+1.3	
	OER	−0.02	−0.01	
Limbic strip	CMRO$_2$	−0.4	0	0.006
	CBF	−0.9	+1.2	
	OER	−0.02	+0.01	

When the neuroleptic-treated psychotic patients were compared with the non-neuroleptic-treated psychotic patients, the treated group generally showed lower rCBF values when compared to the non-treated groups, significant in the frontal and mid-temporal areas on the right side. In these areas the rOER was increased, as it was in the basal ganglia bilaterally. Three patients were evaluated on two occasions either on no neuroleptics or following neuroleptic treatment. Two patients received thioridazine for 1 month, and the third intramuscular fluphenazine. Changes in the rOER, $rCMRO_2$, and rCBF for these patients as a result of treatment are shown in Fig. 6.4. Plate 6.1 demonstrates a rCBF scan of a patient before and after neuroleptic therapy. The patient, who was rated nuclear schizophrenia (NS) on the PSE, had never received neuroleptic medication and had a left temporal focus of abnormality. Following treatment it is possible to see a relative homogenization of the pattern of flow, the laterality differences becoming less marked. Inspection of the data from these patients suggests that the maximum effect noted is on cerebral blood flow, with changes in $rCMRO_2$ being less consistent. The rOER tends to rise reflecting this change of coupling between metabolism and flow.

DISCUSSION

PET scanning has been extremely important in elaborating further some of the cerebral metabolic changes that are seen in patients with epilepsy. Interictally it would appear that patients with primary generalized seizures are likely to show minimal disturbances, but greater and focal changes are seen in those with partial seizures, in particular in patients with a temporal lobe focus where interictal hypometabolism is a constant finding. The hypometabolism is fairly extensive and involves a number of limbic-system-related structures including temporal and frontal cortex and the basal ganglia. These changes do not seem to be directly related to anti-convulsant medication although further studies on the effects of anti-convulsant drugs on cerebral metabolism and blood flow are long overdue. In the study of epileptic psychosis which we have carried out, the metabolic changes seen in non-psychotic patients with temporal lobe epilepsy are also detected but are present to a more significant degree. It is particularly interesting that the temporal areas of the dominant hemisphere appear to be maximally affected in the psychotic patients, while the laterality differences in the non-psychotic control group are less clear. This is in keeping with the substantial literature which suggests that patients with a left-sided temporal lobe focus are more likely when psychotic to present with a schizophreniform presentation (see Trimble 1984). In our study the effect is unlikely to be due to an artefact of more patients in one of the two groups having a temporal lobe focus on the left side, since the groups

---

Fig. 6.4. Changes in rOER (a), $rCMRO_2$ (b), and rCBF (c) in three patients on and off neuroleptic drugs. These indicate how neuroleptic medication tends to decrease the CBF, has less effect upon the $CMRO_2$, resulting in an increase in the OER. Plain, before neuroleptic drugs; speckled, after neuroleptic drugs.

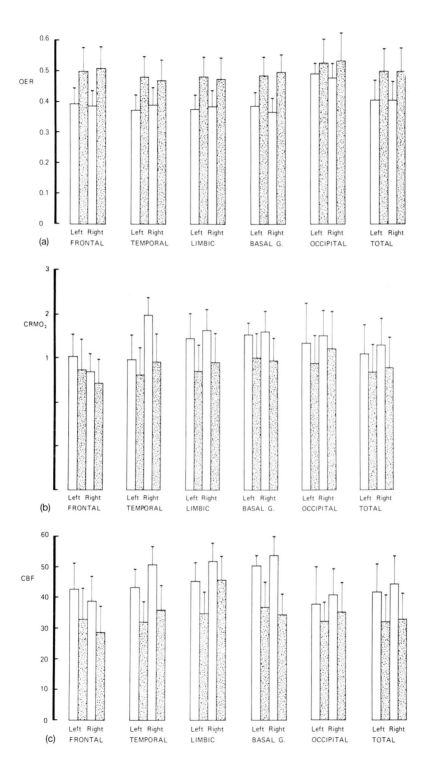

were approximately equal with regards to the laterality of the focus. This finding of a laterality difference in metabolism is particularly important in view of the laterality changes that are now being looked for in PET studies of patients with schizophrenia who do not have epilepsy. Laterality effects have thus been recorded by Shepherd *et al.* (1983), DeLisi *et al.* (1983), and Wolkin *et al.* (1984). However, at the present time there is no clear consistency with these data, for example Shepherd *et al.* (1983) and DeLisi *et al.* (1983) suggesting an increase in metabolic activity in the dominant hemisphere in schizophrenia, while Wolkin *et al.* (1984) note pretreatment schizophrenics to have lower absolute metabolic activity in both frontal and temporal regions, maximal on the left side. In that study, basal ganglia values although lower on the left side, were not significantly different. However, Buchsbaum *et al.* (1983) have reported a significant difference between normal and schizophrenic patients with regards to fluorodeoxyglucose uptake in the central grey mattrer, greater on the left, suggesting hypometabolism in the schizophrenic group.

The epilepsy data are therefore compatible with the findings of psychoses in non-epileptic patients and give support and validity to the concept that the metabolic disturbances somehow reflect on a fundamental biological aspect of the psychoses. The fact that on PET scan studies the area maximally affected in epileptic patients with temporal lobe epilepsy are limbic-system-related and that disturbances of the limbic system are now being described in schizophrenic patients without epilepsy using a variety of techniques emphasizes the importance of the epileptic psychotic model as one method for exploring the pathogenesis of psychosis.

The findings presented here on changes in rCBF and metabolism in patients prescribed neuroleptic medication emphasizes the importance of examining psychotic patients who are neuroleptic-free. Thus, a number of the earlier cerebral blood-flow studies in schizophrenia did not eliminate the possiblity that the findings, particularly those of hypofrontality, were linked to the prolonged prescription of these medications. There seems to be a general effect of these drugs across wide areas of the brain, arguing against a specific locus of action such as the dopamine-rich basal ganglia areas; whether or not this more general effect is linked to their therapeutic proficiency is difficult to comment on with the present state of knowledge, but it is particularly interesting that laterality differences that appear to relate to the presence of psychoses seem minimized following treatment. Our data stand in contrast to those with glucose which suggest that following neuroleptic administration a significant increase in the CMRglucose occurs. Whether this is related to the selection of patients we have chosen (with epilepsy) or is related to some differences between the oxygen and glucose technique is not clear at the present time. Thus it may be that following the administration of such drugs, membrane kinetics are changed leading to alterations in the Sokolof equation, which may lead to the calculation of an apparent metabolic rate for glucose which may then differ from that for oxygen. Clearly further studies noting the different effects of medications using both glucose and oxygen may help elucidate further the fundamental similarities and differences between these techniques for estimating brain metabolism.

REFERENCES

Baron, J. C., Roeda, D., Munari, C., Courzel, C., Stoffels, C., Chodkiewicz, J. P., and Comar, D. (1983). Brain regional pharmacokinetics of 11C-Diphenylhydantoin: Positron Emission Tomography in man. *Neurology* **33**, 580–5.

Bernardi, S., Trimble, M. R., Frackowiak, R. S. J., Wise, R. J. S., and Jones, T. (1983). An interictal study of partial epilepsy using Positron Emission Tomography and the Oxygen-15 inhalation technique. *J. Neurol. Neurosurg. Psychiat.* **46**, 473–7.

Buchsbaum, M. S., Holcomb, H. H., Kessler, R. M., Johnson, J., King, A. C., Cappelletti, J., Bisserbe, J. C., Van Kammen, D. P., Manning, R. J., and Channing, M. (1983). Lateralised asymmetries in glucose up-take assessed by Positron Emission Tomography in patients with schizophrenia and normal controls. In P. Flor-Henry and J. Gruzelier (eds)) *Hemispheric asymmetries of function in psychopathology*, Vol. 2. Elsevier, Amsterdam.

DeLisi, L. E., Buchsbaum, M. S., Irvine, C. A. Dowling, S., Johnson, J., Holcomb, H. H., Kessler, R., and Boronow, J. (1983). Clinical correlates of PET in schizophrenia. New research abstracts. *American Psychiatric Association Annual Meeting, New York*, May 1983. NR 49.

Depresseux, J. C., Franck, G., and Swadzot, B. (1984). Regional cerebral blood flow and oxygen uptake rate in human focal epilepsy. In (eds H. Baldy, M. Moulinier, D. H. Ingvar and B. S. Meldrum), *Current problems in epilepsy, cerebral blood flow, metabolism and epilepsy.* pp. 76–81. John Libbey, London.

Engel, J., Kuhl, D. E., Phelps, M. E., and Maziotta, J. C. (1982*a*). Interictal cerebral glucose metabolism in partial epilepsy and its relation to EEG changes. *Ann. Neurol.* **12**, 518–28.

—— Brown, W. J., Duhl, D. E., Phelps, M. E., Mazziotta, J. C., and Crandall, P. H. (1982*b*). Pathological findings of focal temporal hypometabolism in partial epilepsy. *Ann. Neurol.* **12**, 518–28.

Frackowiak, R. S. J., Lenzi, G. L., Jones, T., and Heather, J. D. (1980). Quantitative measurement of regional cerebral blood flow and oxygen metabolism in man using 15-0 and positron emission tomography: theory, procedure and normal values. *J. Comput. Assist. Tomog.* **4**, 727–36.

Grant, F. C., Spitz, E. G., Shenkin, H. A. (1947). Cerebral blood flow and metabolism in idiopathic epilepsy. *Trans. Amer. Neurol. Ass.* **12**, 82–6.

Gur, R. C., Sussman, N. M., Alavi, A., (1982). Positron Emission Tomography in two cases of childhood epileptic encephalopathy. *Neurology* **32**, 1191–5.

Hill, D. (1953). Psychiatric disorders of epilepsy. *Med. Press.* **229**, 473–5.

Hougaard, K., Oikawa, T., Sveinsdottire, E. (1976). Regional cerebral blood flow in focal cortical epilepsy. *Arch. Neurol.* **33**, 527–35.

Ingvar, D. H. (1975). RCBF in focal cortical epilepsy. In *Cerebral circulation and metabolism* (eds T. W. Langfitt, L. C. McHenry, M. Reivich, and H. Wollman) pp. 361–4. Springer-Verlag, Heidleberg.

Kety, S. S. and Schmidt, C. F. (1948). The nitrous oxide method for determination of cerebral blood flow in man: theory, procedure and normal values. *J. Clin. Invest.* **27**, 476–83.

Lavy, S., Melamed, E., Portnoy, Z., and Carmon, A. (1976). Interictal regional cerebral blood flow in patients with partial seizures. *Neurology* **26**, 418–22.

Mazziotta, J. D. and Engel, J. (1984). The use and impact of positron computed tomography scanning in epilepsy. *Epilepsia* **25**, *Suppl.* **2**, s86–s104.

Penfield, W. and Jasper, H. (1954). *Epilepsy and the functional anatomy of the human brain.* Little Brown and Company, Boston.

Pond, D. A. (1957). Psychiatric aspects of epilepsy. *J. Ind. Med. Prof.* **3**, 1441–51.

Sanabria, E., Chauvel, P., Askienazy, S., Vignal, J. P. (1983). Single photon emission computed tomography using IAMP in partial epilepsy. In (eds. H. Baldy, M. Moulinier, D. H. Ingvar, and B. Meldrum) *Current problems in epilepsy, cerebral blood low, metabolism and epilepsy* pp. 82–5. John Libbey, London.

Shepherd, G., Gruzelier, J., Manchanda, R., Hirsch, S. R., Wise, R., Frackowiak, R. S. J., and Jones, T. (1983). 15-0 Positron Emission Tomographic Scanning in predominantly never treated acute schizophrenic patients. *Lancet* **ii**, 1448–52.

Silverskiöld, P., Gustafson, L., and Risberg, J. (1984). rCBF changes following seizures in two cases of organic affective syndrome. In *Current problems in epilepsy* (eds. M. Baldy, M. Moulinier, D. Ingvar, and B. Meldrum), pp. 39–43. John Libbey, London.

Slater, E. and Beard, A. W. (1963). The schizophrenia-like psychoses of epilepsy. *Brit. J. Psychiat.* **109**, 95–150.

Theodore, W. H., Newark, M. E., and Sato, S. (1983). 18-F Fluorodeoxyglucose positron emission computed tomography in refractory complex partial seizures. *Ann. Neurol.* **14**, 429–43.

Trimble, M. R. (1981). *Neuropsychiatry.* John Wiley, & Sons, Chichester.

—— (1984). Interictal behaviour and temporal lobe epilepsy. *Recent Adv. Epilepsy* **1**, 211–29.

—— Bernardi, S., Gallhofer, B., Frackowiak, R. S. J., Wise, R. J. S., and Jones, T. (1984). An inter-ictal study of partial epilepsy using the oxygen-15 inhalation technique and positron emission tomography, with special reference to psychosis. In *Current problems in epilepsy* (eds. M. Baldy, M. Moulinier, D. Ingvar, and B. Meldrum). Cerebral blood flow, metabolism and epilepsy, pp. 44–50. John Libbey, London.

Wing, J. K., Cooper, J. E., and Sartorius, N. (1974). *The description and classification of psychiatric symptoms.* Cambridge University Press, London.

Wolkin, A., Jaeger, J., and Brodie, J. D. (1984). Persistance of cerebral metabolic abnormalities in chronic schizophrenia as determined by positron emission tomography. *Amer. J. Psychiat.* (in press).

Yamamoto, Y. L., Ochs, R., and Gloor, P. (1984). Patterns of rCBF and focal energy metabolic changes in relation to electroencephalographic abnormality in the interictal phase of partial epilepsy. In *Current problems in epilepsy, cerebral blood flow, metabolism and epilepsy* (eds H. Baldy, M. Moulinier, D. Ingvar, and B. Meldrum), pp. 39–43. John Libbey, London.

7

Cerebral blood flow and metabolism in dementia, with reference to the effects of pharmacological intervention

J. M. GIBBS

INTRODUCTION

The earliest studies of cerebral blood flow and metabolism in dementia were carried out in the 1950s: blood flow was measured by the nitrous oxide technique of Kety and Schmidt (1948), and with a simultaneous record of the arteriovenous oxygen difference across the brain, a global value for cerebral oxygen consumption could be derived (Freyhan *et al.* 1951; Lassen *et al.* 1957). These and later studies demonstrated (not unexpectedly) that both blood flow and metabolic activity are reduced in the brains of demented patients. The subsequent development of methods to measure regional cerebral flow—usually by injection or inhalation of labelled xenon—led to the observation that certain areas of the brain may be affected more severely than others in various types of organic dementia (Ingvar and Gustafson 1970; Obrist *et al.* 1970). Some authors reported a close correlation between the severity of dementia and the degree of reduction of cerebral blood flow (CBF) in certain parts of the brain (Ingvar *et al.* 1968). Others have not been able to show this relationship so clearly (Melamed *et al.* 1978). It has been suggested that the reduction of CBF is more profound in patients with dementia due to vascular disease than in those with degenerative dementia of Alzheimer type (Hachinski *et al.* 1975).

One important question which has been the subject of controversy from the earliest days of CBF measurement is whether attempts to increase cerebral blood flow—by either medical or surgical means—have any place at all in the treatment of patients with dementia. It is generally accepted that the degenerative process underlying Alzheimer's disease is primarily neuronal, and is therefore most unlikely to be influenced by an increase of cerebral blood flow. In the case of dementia due to cerebrovascular disease, however, there is still a surviving view that some patients' symptoms result from a critically low blood flow in certain areas of the brain, and that this ischaemic cerebral dysfunction could theoretically be reversed by improving local CBF. Whether or not this hypothesis is widely accepted, there is still a substantial market for vasoactive drugs which are thought to help demented patients in this way. Some agents can unquestionably be shown to increase CBF in patients with dementia (e.g. Merory *et al.* 1978). However, this type of observation does not confirm that such drugs will either improve an existing neurological deficit or prevent further deterioration of the dementing process. The important consideration is not so much the absolute level of cerebral blood flow as the adequacy of that flow to meet the residual metabolic demands of surviving brain.

The early global measurements of CBF and cerebral oxygen consumption ($CMRO_2$) generally showed a matched reduction of flow and metabolism in dementia (Freyhan *et al.* 1951; Lassen *et al.* 1957). However, the lack of regional data obtained with the Kety–Schmidt technique made it difficult to be certain that there were not some areas of brain receiving a relative excess of blood supply ('luxury perfusion') while flow in other areas was inappropriately low for prevailing metabolic demands (ischaemia).

Measurement of cerebral metabolic activity in a regional manner was first carried out in the 1970s. Grubb and colleagues (1977) used the positron-emitting isotope oxygen-15 with a non-tomographic system of external detectors to assess regional $CMRO_2$ in patients with dementia. However, this technique was limited by relatively low spatial resolution and could not provide reliable quantitative data from deeper structures within the brain. It was the development of computerized tomographic reconstruction technology, at first applied to X-ray imaging of the brain, that finally provided a method for making precise regional measurements of both blood flow and metabolism in the brain. By measuring the local concentration of an appropriate biological tracer at any point within a tomographic slice of brain, positron emission tomography (PET) could display and quantify physiological data in a manner analogous to the reconstruction of an anatomical image by the conventional X-ray (transmission) CT scanner.

The principles and practice of positron tomography have been reviewed extensively elsewhere (Phelps *et al.* 1982; Heiss and Phelps 1983). The technique and some of its applications are discussed at some length in Dr Frackowiak's contribution to this volume (Chapter 2), and will not be dealt with in detail here. However, one crucial advantage of PET over previous techniques requires particular emphasis: this is the capacity to make combined measurements of both the rate of supply of oxygen to the brain (blood flow) and of the level of metabolic demand ($CMRO_2$).

In the normal brain less than half of the oxygen delivered to the tissues in the arterial blood is actually extracted for metabolic consumption, a substantial reserve of oxygen remaining unused. This normally low oxygen extraction of 35–45 per cent is expressed as an oxygen extraction ratio (OER) of 0.35–0.45. The importance of the reserve of unextracted oxygen becomes apparent in states of cerebral ischaemia. Studies in acute stroke have shown that when blood flow is critically reduced in relation to cerebral metabolic demands, oxygen consumption can still be maintained at least partially by a compensatory increase in the fractional extraction of oxygen from what little blood supply remains (Wise *et al.* 1983). In acute ischaemia up to 90 per cent of available arterial oxygen may be extracted in an attempt to maintain normal tissue function (OER = 0.90). The OER is therefore an important expression of the relationship between metabolic supply and demand, representing a quantitative index of the adequacy of existing blood flow to meet the oxygen requirements of surviving tissue. Irrespective of the absolute value of CBF in a particular cerebral region, the finding of a raised OER indicates that prevailing flow is inappropriately low in relation to the local metabolic rate. Conversely, a lower than normal value of regional OER (e.g. 0.20–0.30) indicates that flow is inappropriately high, a situation sometimes referred to as luxury perfusion. The relevance of the OER measurement in the study of dementia is discussed further below, with particular reference to the possible value of increasing CBF in patients with cerebrovascular disease.

With the above background information in mind, the remainder of this chapter will consist of two parts: firstly a brief review of previous PET studies of dementing disorders, and secondly an introduction to some recent studies investigating the effects of a vasoactive drug in patients with dementia resulting from vascular disease.

PET STUDIES IN DEMENTIA

The first (and still the most comprehensive) study of cerebral blood flow and metabolism in dementia was that of Frackowiak *et al.* (1981), in which both clinical and detailed physiological data were reported from 22 patients, 13 with presumed degenerative pathology and 9 with dementia attributed to cerebrovascular disease. The clinical severity of dementia was graded from a standard neuropsychological scoring system (Blessed *et al.* 1968), supplemented by assessment of specific focal deficits such as dysphasia and constructional apraxia in each case. In general, the degree of reduction of CBF and $CMRO_2$ was found to correlate quite closely with the severity of dementia in both the degenerative and vascular patient groups. Not unexpectedly, the distribution of hypometabolism in the vascular cases was often asymmetrical and showed marked variation from case to case, in keeping with the patchy cerebral damage that results from multi-infarct disease. A typical example of this is shown in Plate 7.1, the PET images from a relatively young woman with a history of stepwise intellectual deterioration occurring in the context of a systemic vasculitic disorder.

Amongst the patients with degenerative dementia of Alzheimer type, early cases were characterized by most marked reduction of CBF and $CMRO_2$ in the parietal and temporal regions of both cerebral hemispheres. More advanced degenerative dementia was associated with profound functional depression also in the frontal regions. In all cases there was a matched reduction of CBF and $CMRO_2$ (OER normal), indicating that flow was appropriately low in response to diminished cerebral metabolic demands. Even amongst the vascular cases there were no regions of increased OER, supporting the widely held belief that the dementia in such cases results from multiple established infarcts, rather than from a state of continuing (and potentially reversible) cerebral ischaemia.

Benson and colleagues (1983) measured regional cerebral glucose metabolism in eleven patients with dementia, eight with Alzheimer's disease, and three with multiple cerebral infarcts. As in Franckowiak's study, those with degenerative dementia showed a symmetrical pattern of hypometabolism, mainly affecting the parietal, temporal, and frontal areas, while cases of multi-infarct disease were characterized by more patchy and asymmetrical abnormalities. These authors stressed the fact that the primary motor, sensory, and visual cortical areas were relatively spared in their patients with Alzheimer's disease, consistent with the typical pattern of clinical involvement in this disorder. The degree of reduction of metabolism observed in this study was profound, mean cerebral glucose consumption (CMRG1c) being 49 per cent lower in demented patients than in age-matched controls. In an earlier report by Alavi *et al.* (1981), who also measured CMRG1c by the fluorine-18 fluorodeoxyglucose method, a more modest reduction of 20–30 per cent was observed in demented subjects.

Chase and colleagues (1984) have reported an overall 30 per cent reduction of CMRG1c in 17 patients with dementia of Alzheimer type. These authors drew attention to the regional bias of the abnormalities in their patients with Alzheimer's disease, the most marked metabolic depression being noted in the posterior parietal and temporal regions of both cerebral hemispheres, with relative sparing of the frontal lobes. This pattern corresponded closely to the deficit in oxygen consumption and blood flow observed in less severely demented patients by Frackowiak *et al.* (1981). Chase and co-workers also found that specific neuropsychological deficits in individual patients could usually be correlated with a marked focal reduction of glucose consumption in the appropriate region of the brain. Those with disproportionate language disturbance all showed conspicuous hypometabolism in the left parasylvian region; those with severe visual spatial dysfunction consistently had a focus of low metabolic activity in the right posterior parietal region; features of Gerstmann's syndrome apparently correlated with hypometabolism around the angular gyrus; and marked personality deterioration in some patients was associated with more severe frontal lobe involvement. Observations of this kind are of some academic interest, reinforcing existing knowledge about localization of function in the brain and highlighting the subtle variability of focal involvement in different patients with Alzheimer's disease. However, it cannot be said that such studies have added substantially to our understanding of the nature of the disease itself.

Tracer techniques are also being developed for the study of protein metabolism in the brain. Bustany *et al.* (1983) have described a model using PET with carbon-11-labelled methionine for the measurement of regional amino acid incorporation, an index of cerebral protein synthesis. Studies of patients with Alzheimer's disease have shown marked reduction of labelled methionine uptake, values in severely demented patients being anything up to 65 per cent lower than those in normal subjects (Bustany *et al.* 1983). These changes were found to be most marked in the frontal lobes, although as with the measurement of oxygen and glucose metabolism, the parietal association areas were also affected to some degree.

Another degenerative disorder in which PET studies have been of particular interest is Huntington's chorea. Kuhl and co-workers (1984), applying the fluorodeoxyglucose technique to measure cerebral glucose metabolism, have studied patients with varying degrees of dementia and movement disorder. A characteristic pattern was observed in which CMRG1c was focally reduced in the caudate nuclei and putaminal regions. This hypometabolism was clearly detectable even in patients with relatively mild disease in whom the characteristic X-ray CT scan appearances had not yet developed. Typically, glucose utilization was found to be normal throughout the rest of the brain, regardless of the severity of symptoms and despite the presence of structural cortical atrophy on the CT scans in many cases. Furthermore, preliminary results suggest that hypometabolism in the caudate nuclei may be detectable in potential cases of Huntington's disease even when these subjects are still entirely asymptomatic. This observation highlights the sensitivity of the technique and implies that such studies could be of considerable practical value in the management and counselling of families affected by this distressing condition.

PHARMACOLOGICAL INTERVENTION IN PATIENTS WITH MULTI-INFARCT DEMENTIA

Although the concept of chronic cerebral ischaemia dies hard, there is increasingly wide acceptance of the view that the dementia of cerebrovascular disease results from an accumulation of multiple, irreversible ischaemic lesions in the brain. Hypertensive lacunar infarcts are probably the most common pathological substrate of multi-infarct dementia, while more peripheral lesions resulting from multiple embolic occlusions of larger vessels account for a minority of cases (Pearce 1978). A predominantly intellectual deficit may also result from 'haemodynamic' cerebral infarction involving mutliple watershed areas of the brain (Pearce 1978). This type of lesion may result from a single catastrophic hypotensive episode in patients with normal cerebral vessels, but is also characteristic of occlusive extracranial arterial disease, particularly when cerebral perfusion pressure is profoundly reduced by occlusion of two or more of the major neck vessels (Romanul and Abramowicz 1964).

Control of hypertension and prevention of further cerebral emboli are important palliative measures in some patients with multi-infarct dementia. What is much less certain is whether therapeutic measures to increase cerebral perfusion have any value in the treatment of dementia due to vascular disease. The earlier PET findings of Frackowiak *et al.* (1981) suggested that the low CBF in demented patients is entirely appropriate for the reduced metabolic requirements of damaged brain, and that any increase of blood flow would be redundant in these cases. A recent study at the Hammersmith Hospital set out to examine the effects of a vasoactive drug on cerebral blood flow and metabolism in patients with multi-infarct dementia.

In 14 patients with dementia, a presumptive diagnosis of multi-infarct disease was based on the clinical features incorporated in the Ishaemia Score of Hachinski *et al.* (1975), supported in most but not all cases by appropriate abnormalities on the CT scan. Regional CBF, CMRO$_2$, and OER were measured by PET, using the oxygen-15 steady-state technique (Frackowiak *et al.* 1981; see also Chapter 2). Studies through identical tomographic planes were made in each patient before and after intravenous administration of a vasodilator drug, the patients remaining undisturbed on the scanning couch throughout the period of study. In eight of the 14 patients there was no significant change of CBF, CMRO$_2$, or OER after drug administration. In the remaining six cases a transient rise of CBF was observed. This increase of flow was not accompanied by any change of cerebral function as judged by regional oxygen consumption. Since CBF rose and CMRO$_2$ remained unchanged, there was a reciprocal fall of OER in each case. The quantitative results from these six patients are summarized in Figure 7.1, the values shown being the mean from several standardized regions of interest in both cerebral hemispheres. Plate 7.2 shows the physiological images from one of the six cases. Note the slight generalised rise of CBF, with a reciprocal fall of OER, observed only in the first of the two tomographic planes studied

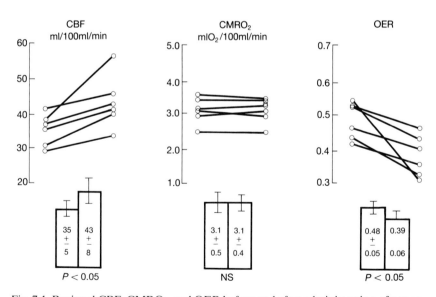

Fig. 7.1. Regional CBF, CMRO$_2$, and OER before and after administration of a vasodilator drug. Note the unchanged CMRO$_2$ and the reciprocal fall of OER in all cases. (Statistical comparisons by paired *t*-test.)

(third column of images from the left); this indicated that the effect of the drug on CBF was evident only during the first 5 min after administration (the time taken to carry out the blood flow scan of the first tomographic plane).

The important point was that the pretreatment blood flow in these patients was already apparently adequate (CBF appropriately matched to $CMRO_2$, OER normal), and the increase of flow was not associated with any increase of cerebral metabolic activity. Because the additional flow was redundant, the brain adjusted by extracting a smaller proportion of the available oxygen than before (39 per cent as opposed to 48 per cent in the group of six patients as a whole). Careful analysis of numerous regions in the brains of these patients revealed no areas of true ischaemia, in which CBF was critically low before treatment and then rose to a more appropriate level after administration of the drug. In fact from what is known about the mechanism of auto-regulation, such a state of ischaemia should already be associated with maximal vasodilation in the affected region and it would be surprising if a locally active drug could then increase CBF above its existing level.

The above observations, although limited to a very small number of cases, clearly support the view that there is little to be gained by increasing CBF in patients with multi-infarct dementia.

To put these results fully into perspective, two additional points should be made. First, it must not be assumed that pharmacological enhancement of cerebral function will invariably be accompanied by a detectable increase of metabolic activity in some part of the brain. For example, dramatic clinical improvement following L -dopa administration in patients with Parkinson's disease has been shown to occur without any change of $CMRO_2$ in the basal ganglia or elsewhere (Leenders *et al.* 1985). Secondly, there are occasional patients with dementia resulting from vascular disease in whom there *is* a critical reduction of CBF in relation to cerebral metabolic demands. This situation, in which there is focal elevation of OER in the ischaemic region, is encountered in a small minority of patients with widespread occlusive disease of the carotid and vertebral arteries (Baron *et al.* 1981; Gibbs *et al.* 1984). In cases of this sort, further episodes of infarction in the watershed areas of the brain may theoretically be prevented by appropriate surgical measures to improve cerebral perfusion pressure in the ischaemic areas of the brain. It should be stressed, however, that only a very small minority of patients with multi-infarct dementia are likely to fall into this 'haemodynamic' category.

SUMMARY

Numerous PET studies have confirmed the observations made by pioneering workers using earlier, more invasive techniques: namely, that both cerebral blood flow and metabolism are consistently reduced in patients with organic dementia of various types. Useful information about the regional pattern of these abnormalities has been added to the global measurements obtained by original techniques. In all cases of degenerative dementia and the vast majority of those with multi-infarct disease, CBF is appropriately reduced in relation to the diminished metabolic requirements of damaged brain. Attempts to increase cerebral blood flow by pharmacological means are most unlikely to bring about any improvement of cerebral function in such cases. In a small minority of patients with dementia associated with occlusive carotid artery disease, further deterioriation may possibly be prevented by direct carotid or transcranial bypass surgery.

Positron emission tomography should continue to be a valuable research tool in the evaluation of local vascular and metabolic effects of drugs designed to influence cerebral function in degenerative neurological disorders.

REFERENCES

Alavi, A., Ferris, S., and Wolf, A. (1981). Determination of cerebral metabolism in senile dementia using F-18-deoxyglucose and positron tomography (Abstract). *J. Nucl. Med.* **21**, 21.

Baron, J. C., Bousser, M. G., Rey, A., Guillard, A., Comar, D., and Castaigne, P. Reversal of 'misery perfusion syndrome' by extra-intracranial arterial bypass in haemodynamic cerebral ischaemia. *Stroke* **12**, 454–9.

Benson, D. F., Kuhl, D. E., Hawkins, R. A., Phelps, M. E., Cummings, J. L., and Tsai, S. Y. (1983). The fluorodeoxyglucose ^{18}F scan in Alzheimer's disease and multi-infarct dementia. *Arch. Neurol.* **40**, 711–14.

Blessed, G.,Tomlinson, B. E., and Roth, M. (1968). The association between quantitative measures of dementia and of senile change in the cerebral grey matter of elderly demented subjects. *Br. J. Psychiat.* **114**, 797–811.

Bustany, P., Henry, J. F., Sargent, T., Zarifian, E., Cabanis, E., Collard, P., and Comar, D. (1983). Local brain protein metabolism in dementia and schizophrenia: *in vivo* studies with 11-C-L-methionine and positron emission tomography. In *Positron emission tomography of the brain* (eds W.-D. Heiss and M. E. Phelps), Springer-Verlag, New York. pp. 208–11.

Chase, T, N., Foster, N. L., Fedio, P., Brooks, R., Mansi, L., and Di Chiro, G. (1984). Regional cortical dysfunction in Alzheimer's disease as determined by positron emission tomography. *Ann. Neurol.* **15** (Supl.), S170–4.

Frackowiak, R. S. J., Pozzilli, C., Legg, N. J., Du Boulay, G. H., Marshall, J., Lenzi, G. L., and Jones, T. (1981). Regional cerebral oxygen supply and utilisation in dementia: a clinical and physiological study with oxygen-15 and positron tomography. *Brain* **104**, 753–78.

Freyhan, F. A., Woodford, R. B., and Kety, S. S. (1951). Cerebral blood flow and metabolism in psychoses of senility. *J. Nerv. Ment. Dis.* **113**, 449–56.

Gibbs, J. M., Wise, R. J. S., Leenders, K. L., and Jones, T. (1984). Evaluation of cerebral perfusion reserve in patients with carotid artery occlusion. *Lancet* **1**, 310–14.

Grubb, R. L., Raichle, M. E., Gado, M. H., Eichling, J. O., and Hughes, C. P. (1977). Cerebral blood flow, oxygen utilisation and blood volume in dementia. *Neurology (Minneap).* **27**, 95–10.

Hachinski, V. C., Iliff, L. D., Zilkha, E., Du Boulay, G. H., McAllister, V. L., Marshall, J., Ross Russell, R. W., and Symon, L. (1975). Cerebral blood flow in dementia. *Arch. Neurol. (Chic)* **32**, 632–7.

Heiss, W. D., and Phelps, M. E. (eds) (1983). *Positron emission tomography of the brain.* Springer-Verlag, New York.

Ingvar, D. H. and Gustafson, LO. (1970). Regional cerebral blood flow in organic dementia of early onset. *Acta Neurol. Scand.* **46** (*Suppl.* **43**), 42–73.

Kety, S. S. and Schmidt, E. F. (1948). The nitrous oxide method for determination of cerebral blood flow in man: theory, procedure and normal values. *J. Clin. Invest.* **27**, 476–83.

Kuhl, D. E., Metter, E. J., Riege, W. H., and Markham, C. H. (1984). Patterns of cerebral glucose utilization in Parkinson's disease and Huntingdon's disease. *Ann. Neurol.* **15** (Suppl.), 5119–25.

Lassen, N. A., Munck, O., and Tottey, E. R. (1957). Mental function and cerebral oxygen consumption in organic dementia. *Arch. Neurol. Psychiat. (Chic)* **77**, 126–33.

Leenders, K. L., Wolfson, L., Gibbs, J. M., Wise, R. J. S., Causon, R., Jones, T., and Legg, N. J. (1985). The effects of L -Dopa on regional cerebral blood flow and oxygen metabolism in patients with Parkinson's disease. *Brain* (in press).

Melamed, E., Lavy, S., Siew, F., Bentin, S., and Cooper, G. (1978). Correlation between regional cerebral blood flow and brain atrophy in dementia. *J. Neurol. Neurosurg. Psychiat.* **41**, 894–9.

Merory, J., Du Boulay, G. H., Marshall, J., Morris, J., Ross Russell, R. W., Symon, L., and Thomas, D. J. (1978). Effect of tinofedrine (Homburg D8955) on cerebral blood flow in multi-infarct dementia. *J. Neurol. Neurosurg. Psychiat.* **41**, 9002–2.

Obrist, W. D., Chivian, E., Cronquist, S., and Ingvar, D. H. (1970). Regional cerebral blood flow in senile and pre-senile dementia. *Neurology* **20**, 315–22.

Pearce, J. M. S. (1978). Dementia in cerebral arterial disease. In *Vascular disease of the central nervous system* (ed. R. W. Ross Russell)., Churchill Livingstone, London.

Phelps, M. E., Mazziotta, J. C., and Huang, S. C. (1982). Study of cerebral function with positron computed tomography. *J. Cereb. Blood. Flow. Metab.* **2**, 113–62.

Romanul, F. C. A. and Abramowicz, A. (1964). Changes in brain and pial vessels in arterial border zones. *Arch. Neurol. (Chic.)* **11**, 40–65.

Wise, R. J. S., Bernardi, S., Frackowiak, R. S. J., Legg, N. J., and Jones, T. (1983). Serial observations on the pathophysiology of acute stroke: the transition from ischaemia to infarction as reflected in regional oxygen extraction. *Brain* **106**, 197–222.

8

Regional cerebral blood flow and depression: an application of the ^{133}Xe inhalation method

P. UYTDENHOEF, J. JACQUY, AND J. MENDLEWICZ

INTRODUCTION

Several studies in different fields (genetics, biochemistry, neuroendocrinology, neurophysiology, chronobiology) have reported biological abnormalities in patients with affective disorders, suggesting that at least some subtypes of depression are related to biological cerebral dysfunction. Using different techniques, such as skin conductance measurement, EEG, and PET scan, some authors have found differential hemispheric and regional involvement in affective disorders. Most of them have reported a relative left hemispheric deactivation (Myslobodsky and Horesh 1978; D'Elia and Perris 1973; Phelps *et al.* 1983) but other authors have found abnormalities in the right (Flor-Henry 1976) or in both hemispheres (Perris and Monakhov 1979; Mathew *et al.* 1980).

Since that cerebral blood flow is tightly coupled to cerebral metabolism and function (Raichle *et al.* 1976), some authors have studied the regional cerebral blood flow (rCBF) in depression.

THE ^{133}Xe INHALATION TECHNIQUE

The ^{133}Xe inhalation technique for rCBF measurement is non-invasive, reliable, and reproducible (Obrist *et al.* 1975; Meyer *et al.* 1978). ^{133}Xe, a chemically inert and diffusible gas which emits gamma activity, is mixed with ambient air and inhaled through a face mask. After a 1-min period of inhalation, the decreasing activity of the isotope is monitored for 10 min by 16 collimated probes, mounted in a helmet and applied to the scalp. The end-tidal ^{133}Xe radioactivity is also measured. The values of rCBF are calculated by two compartmental analyses of the recorded curves, by a computer during the 10-min desaturation period. This analysis is based on the Fick principle, and the end-tidal ^{133}Xe curves, recorded from the face mask, are used for correction of ^{133}Xe recirculation to the brain. Table 8.1 shows the limits and advantages of the ^{133}Xe inhalation method.

INVESTIGATIONS

In a first study (Schittecatte *et al.* 1983), we found significantly decreased global CBF in patients with major depression, when compared to normal

TABLE 8.1. *Limits and advantages of the* ^{133}Xe *inhalation method.*

Limits
> Poor spatial resolution
> Recirculation of the tracer
> Extracerebral contamination
> Indirect index of metabolism
> Usually non-tomographic

Advantages
> Non-invasive
> Low irradiation → possible serial measurements
> Relatively inexpensive, available for many centres → contributive clinical use

controls, global CBF improving after recovery. Patients with primary degenerative dementia also showed lower global CBF values. These results are shown in Fig. 8.1.

Because absolute values of CBF can be influenced by non-specific factors like age, vigilance, or P_{CO_2} variations, we preferred to study relative regional values compared with the global CBF of the patients. In a recent study (Uytdenhoef *et al.* 1983*a*), we selected four groups of subjects according to the Research Diagnostic Criteria (Spitzer *et al.* 1975): 16 patients (three men and 13 women; mean age $\pm$ S.D. $= 51.5 \pm 13.4$ years) with the diagnosis of

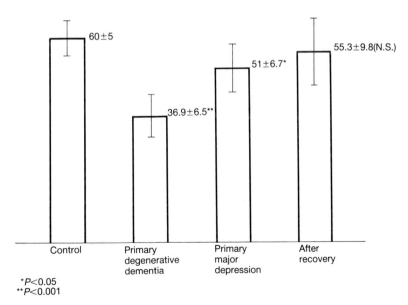

*P<0.05
**P<0.001

Fig. 8.1. Global CBF values in patients with major depression and after recovery, and patients with primary degenerative dementia. The initial slope index (ISI) 2.5 was used.

major depressive disorder; ten patients (three men and seven women; mean age ± S.D. = 35.4 ± 8.1 years) suffering from a minor depression; eight bipolar manic-depressive patients (two men and six women; mean age ± S.D. = 50.6 ± 11 years) studied in a normothymic phase; and 20 non-psychiatric healthy volunteers (eight men and 12 women; mean age ± S.D. = 41 ± 11 years) as a control group. Patients with dementia, migraine, epilepsy, alcoholism, drug addiction, or somatic disorders were excluded from this study through physical examination, EEG, CAT scan, and laboratory tests.

All depressive patients were inpatients and underwent a medication washout period of at least 15 days, except for a benzodiazepine at low dosage (lorazepam, 2.5–7.5 mg/day; mean : 6.7 ± 1.3 for the group of major depressives; mean : 6.6 ± 1.4 for the group of minor depressives; no significant difference).

All manic-depressive patients in remission were treated with lithium carbonate (plasma levels : 0.8–1.4 meq/l) on an outpatient basis, but did not receive any other psychotropic drug for at least 1 month before the study. The severity of depression was quantified by the Hamilton Rating Scale for Depression (Hamilton 1960) on the day of the CBF measurement.

To calculate and interpret the results, we used the initial slope index 2.5 (ISI 2.5), which is the most reliable one with this technique (Prohovnik *et al.* 1980). We expressed each value as a relative one, compared with the global cerebral blood flow of the patient. The four anterior and three posterior probes of each hemisphere were grouped so as to study the frontal and posterior (parieto-temporo-occipital) regions. The different values were then compared, using Student's *t* test and an analysis of variance. Table 8.2 shows the main results of this study. The comparison is between the different groups for frontal and posterior ratios of each hemisphere to the global cerebral blood flow, and for the hemispheric ratio (left/right).

In the group of major depressives, relative values of rCBF were found significantly increased in the left frontal region and significantly decreased in the

TABLE 8.2. *Comparison between the groups of major depression (M), minor depression (m), normothymic bipolar patients (BP), and normal subjects (N). (Relative values of ISI 2.5.)*

	M–N	m–N	BP–N	M–m	M–BP
Left frontal ratio	6.78*	2.24	−1.91	4.54	8.69**
Right frontal ratio	−3.03	1.02	−1.15	−4.05*	−1.88
Left posterior ratio	−0.22	1.72	−0.40	−1.94	0.18
Right posterior ratio	−4.69*	−0.47	1.68	−4.22	−6.37**
Hemispheric ratio (left/right)	6.45	1.45	1.45	5	5

* $P < 0.05$.
** $P < 0.01$.

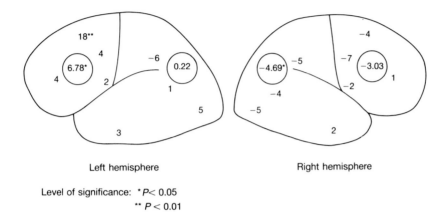

Left hemisphere   Right hemisphere

Level of significance: *$P < 0.05$
** $P < 0.01$

Fig. 8.2. Difference between the group of major depressives and the control group of normal subjects. (Relative values of ISI 2.5.)

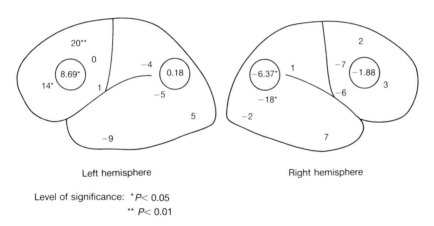

Left hemisphere   Right hemisphere

Level of significance: *$P < 0.05$
** $P < 0.01$

Fig. 8.3. Difference between the group of major depressives and the group of normo-thymic bipolar patients. (Relative values of ISI 2.5.)

right posterior region, when compared to normal controls and to normo-thymic bipolar patients. These relationships were not found with minor depressives or with normothymic bipolar patients. The differences are also illustrated in Figs. 8.2 and 8.3. Because these abnormalities were not found in bipolar patients in remission, they seem to be state-dependent rather than trait-dependent. The fact that relative values of rCBF return to normal after recovery (Uytdenhoef *et al.* 1983*b*) seems to confirm that the rCBF dis-turbances observed during major depressive episodes are state-dependent.

REVIEW OF THE LITERATURE AND DISCUSSION

There are few CBF studies that have been performed in the field of affective disorders and their results are controversial, at least partly for methodological reasons. First, the use of different diagnostic criteria (Research Diagnostic Criteria, DSM III criteria, etc.) for selecting and excluding patients can partially explain apparently contradictory results. Secondly, the measurement of cerebral blood flow—mainly absolute values—can be influenced by several non-specific factors. Table 8.3 shows some of these.

TABLE 8.3.
*Non-specific factors
affecting CBF values.*

Age
P_{CO_2}
Vigilance
Handedness
Medication
Cerebral diseases
Performing conditions
Intelligence? Sex? Anxiety?

Mathew *et al.* (1980) found decreased absolute CBF values in depressed patients, in the left hemisphere mainly, but did not report P_{CO_2} levels. Gustafson *et al.* (1981) found hemispheric mean flows lower than those of normal subjects but they noted that when differences in age and P_{CO_2} were compensated for, the flow differences between depressives and normals became uncertain. Rush *et al.* (1982) reported bilaterally decreased blood flow in endogenous unipolar depressives, but this study was not controlled for P_{CO_2}, medication, and age effects. In a recent study where P_{CO_2} levels, age, sex, years of education and handedness were controlled, Gur *et al.* (1984) found abnormalities only in activation patterns during cognitive tasks in depressives but no abnormalities in absolute values of CBF in resting conditions in these patients. Nevertheless this study was performed with medicated patients. Using regional analysis, these authors found a relative left frontal overactivation for resting flows in depressive patients, a finding apparently in contradiction to the hypothesis of left hemispheric relative deactivation in depression but consistent with our results. In conclusion, considering the advantages of the ^{133}Xe inhalation method, rCBF studies can surely contribute to investigation of the physiopathology of affective disorders, but a rigorous methodology is essential if we are to detect specific biological phenomena underlying depression.

REFERENCES

D'Elia, G. and Perris, C. (1973). Cerebral functional dominance and depression. *Acta Psychiat. Scand.* **49**, 191–7.

Flor-Henry, P. (1976). Lateralized temporal—limbic dysfunction and psychopathology. *Ann. N.Y. Acad. Sci.* **280**, 777–95.

Gur, R. E., Skolnick, B. E., Gur, R. C., Caroff, S., Rieger, W., Obrist, W. D., Younkin, D., and Reivich, M. (1984). Brain function in psychiatric disorders. *Arch. Gen. Psychiat.* **41**, 695–9.

Gustafson, L., Risberg, J., and Silfverskiold, P. (1981). Regional cerebral blood flow in organic dementia and affective disorders. *Adv. Biol. Psychiat.* **6**, 109–16.

Hamilton, M. (1960). A rating scale for depression. *J. Neurol. Neurosurg. Psychiat.* **23**, 56–62.

Mathew, R. J., Meyer, J. S., Francis, D. J., Semchuk, K. M., Mortel, K., and Claghorn, J. L. (1980). Cerebral blood flow in depression. *Am. J. Psychiat.* **137(11)**, 1449–50.

Meyer, J. S., Ishiara, N., Deshmukh, V. D., Naritomi, H., Sakai, F., Hsu, M. C., and Pollack, P. (1978). Improved method for noninvasive measurement of regional cerebral blood flow by ^{133}Xenon inhalation, Part 1. *Stroke* **9**, 195–204.

Myslobodsky, M. S. and Horesh, N. (1978). Bilateral electrodermal activity in depressive patients. *Biol. Psychiat.* **6**, 111–20.

Obrist, W. D., Thomson, H. K., Wang, H. S., and Wilkinson, W. E. (1975). Regional cerebral blood flow estimated by ^{133}Xenon inhalation. *Stroke* **6**, 245–56.

Perris, C. and Monakhov, K. (1979). Depressive symptomatology and systemic analysis of the EEG. In *Hemisphere asymmetries of function in psychopathology* (eds J. Gruzelier and P. Flor-Henry), pp. 223–36. Elsevier–North-Holland, Biomedical Press, Amsterdam.

Phelps, M., Mazziota, J., Gerner, R., Baxter, L., and Kuhl, D. (1983). Human cerebral glucose metabolism in affective disorders: drug-free states and pharmacological effects. *Cereb. Blood Flow Metab.* **3**, (*Suppl.* **1**), S7–8.

Prohovnik, I., Hakansson, K., and Risberg, J. (1980). Observations on the functional significance of regional cerebral blood flow in 'resting' normal subjects. *Neuropsychologia* **18**, 203–17.

Raichle, M., Grubb, R., Gado, M., Shaw, T., Eichling, J., and Ter Pogossian, M. (1976). Correlation between regional cerebral blood flow and oxidative metabolism. *Arch. Neurol.* **33**, 523–6.

Rush, A. J., Schlesser, M. A., Stokely, E., Bonte, F., and Altshuller, K. (1982). Cerebral blood flow in depression and mania. *Psychopharmacol. Bull.* **18(3)**, 6–8.

Schittecatte, M., Charles, G., Uytdenhoef, P., Jacquy, J., and Wilmotte, J. (1983). Sleep, cerebral blood flow and endogenous depression. *First international symposium of the Belgian association for the study of sleep*, Bruxelles.

Spitzer, R. L., Endicott, J., and Robbins, E. (1975). *Research diagnostic criteria for a selected group of functional disorders* (2nd ed). New York State Psychiatric Institute, New York.

Uytdenhoef, P., Charles, G., Jacquy, J., Portelange, P., Linkowski, P., and Mendlewicz, J. (1983a). Regional cerebral blood flow and lateralized hemispheric dysfunction in depression. *Brit. Psychiat.* **143**, 128–32.

—— Portelange, P., Schittecatte, M., Mendlewicz, J., Wilmotte, J., and Jacquy, J. (1983b). Regional cerebral blood flow in major depression and after recovery. *VIIe Congrès Mondial de Psychiatrie*, Vienne.

9

Nuclear magnetic resonance spectroscopy—future technical prospects

L. D. HALL, S. L. LUCK, T. NORWOOD, V. RAJANAYAGAM, AND J. SCHACHTER

During the decade 1973–1983, and especially during the period, 1980–1983, a series of major technical developments in nuclear magnetic resonance (NMR) transformed this already powerful scientific tool into an equally powerful clinical imaging modality. By far the major emphasis, both commercially and in terms of clinical practice, was directed towards proton tomography. This is now firmly established in many clinical locations around the world as a method for anatomical imaging and, under favourable circumstances, for detecting aberrant pathology. We shall not be directly concerned with that topic in this Chapter although, as we shall see, some of the techniques of tomography can now be adapted for other purposes which are pertinent to the present discussion.

Independently of 'tomography', it was demonstrated in a few laboratories that NMR spectroscopy has substantial potential as a non-invasive, analytical tool for measuring quantitatively *in vivo* levels of certain basic biochemicals. Because this particular area is now attracting substantial attention it seems highly probable that it too is destined to undergo a major revolution. It is the purpose of this Chapter to attempt to anticipate the probable form of that revolution, at least from a technical standpoint.

Anticipating the details, it is clear that it is now possible, in principle at least, to obtain high-resolution NMR spectra from any defined volume within the human body. The excitement engendered by this prospect must be tempered with the harsh realities associated with the low intrinsic sensitivity of the NMR method. Those realities are crudely summarized in the equation:

$$S/N \propto [c](d)^3(t)^{\frac{1}{2}}nB_0$$

and it is instructive to evaluate the parameters involved before we consider the methods used for the point-selective determination of spectra.

The effective signal-to-noise ratio (S/N) is directly proportional to the concentration, $[c]$, of the species of interest. Thus, a 10-fold decrease in concentration results in a 10-fold reduction in S/N. The effect of the spatial resolution chosen for a particular measurement is even more dramatic. Suppose the object of interest to be subdivided into cubes, of side d, and consider the effect of demanding a 10-fold increase in resolution for *each* dimension; this corresponds to a 1000-fold decrease in volume and hence to a 1000-fold decrease in S/N.

Given that for most *in vivo* measurements the concentration of the species of interest is fixed, what recourse does the operator have to overcome an unacceptably low S/N ratio? First the ratio can be increased by accepting data from a suitably large volume of tissue; however, beyond a certain point the resultant loss of spatial definition makes nonsense of the measurement. Alternatively the ratio can be increased by repeatedly sampling the magnetization of the species of interest. Because the noise level increases proportional to the square root of the number (n) of scans, the S/N ratio is proportional to $\sqrt{n}$, and hence to the square root of time (t). Although this is not a high power factor, its implications are non-trivial. Time-averaging to increase the S/N ratio by 10-fold, requires a 100-fold increase in time. The third source of improved S/N ratio stems from an increase in the magnetic field strength (B_0) at which the measurement is made. Because the probe technology used at different frequencies is so different, it is not possible to predict with any accuracy the precise relationship, so it is assumed here that it is linear; almost certainly, future developments will ensure that this is an underestimate, and hence will increasingly favour measurements made at higher field strengths (frequencies).

The choice of nuclear species which is to be studied is the final consideration which has a profound influence on the concentration of the species which can be studied in unit time. The situation is summarized in Table 9.1,

TABLE 9.1. *List of some commonly occurring nuclides which can be detected by NMR.*

Nuclide	Intrinsic sensitivity	Natural abundance (%)	Effective sensitivity
^1H	100.0	100.00	100.0
^{13}C	1.59	1.1	0.018
^{19}F	83.4	100.00	83.4
^{23}Na	9.24	100.00	9.27
^{31}P	6.64	100.00	6.64

which lists the relative *intrinsic* sensitivities of the different 'magnetic' nuclides, together with the *effective* sensitivities if their resonances are studied in natural abundance. Three points merit particular comment. First, the sensitivity of proton NMR is so far in excess of that of the other endogenous chemical species in brain that it simply has to have a unique rôle in future neurological studies. Second, of all the exogenous 'labels' which can be used for labelling studies, ^{19}F is by far the most sensitive. Finally, although ^{13}C has a low effective sensitivity, use of enriched compounds offers a substantial improvement; the implications of that fact will be explored later.

A final technical consideration which merits discussion at this juncture concerns the 'dynamic range' of the NMR measurement. Simply, it is extremely difficult to measure the NMR signal from a species present in low concentration when the sample also has another NMR signal which is very intense, that from water, for example. As we shall see later this has important implications for proton NMR spectroscopic studies of brain metabolites.

The reason for expending so much effort on this seemingly unexciting arithmetic is that although the S/N ratio of NMR spectroscopy is high for the proton resonances of species such as water and fat, it is low for virtually all other NMR measurements which are of interest in brain studies. As a result, many potentially important NMR experiments will require heroic efforts, and many of the most exciting will, unfortunately, never be possible. In what follows, we shall attempt to summarize the methods which have already been developed for determining point-specific NMR spectra from locations within an object, and mention some concepts which may be important in the future.

Much of the pioneering work for *in vivo* NMR spectroscopy was performed in Oxford by the groups of Radda and Richards and by the Oxford Research Systems group. Crucial to all studies was, and continues to be, the availability of magnets based on superconducting selenoids, which were also pioneered in Oxford, by Oxford Instruments. These provide magnetic fields which are of high magnitude and overall homogeneity; the former ensures that the resonance signals from individual species are dispersed in frequency space and the latter that their line widths are as small as possible, which further enhances the resolution of the resonances. From the clinical standpoint the important breakthrough came with the availability of magnets large enough (30 cm bore) to enable spectroscopy to be performed on a human limb, and with a volume of homogeneous field equivalent to a sphere, diameter 4 cm. Operating at a field strength of 1.9 Tesla these gave adequate spectral dispersion and resolution for studies to be made of proton, phosphorus, and carbon spectra. A copy of such spectra is shown in Fig. 9.1.

Given the need to further localize the volume of tissue from which the spectrum was derived, two additional techniques were developed. The first of these involved (Ackerman *et al.* 1980) the use of a 'surface-coil'; instead of placing the sample inside the radiofrequency coil as would be customary for a chemical measurement, a small coil, 2–4 cm diameter, was placed on the external surface of the object. It was then assumed that the depth of penetration of the radiofrequency into the tissue was equal to the diameter of the coil used and that this defined the volume which produced the spectrum. In a subsequent development, 'field-profiling' was used (Gordon *et al.* 1980) to further define the volume within the magnet which could produce a homogeneous field.

This combination enabled a number of important studies to be made. The most important of these involved (Ross *et al.* 1981) measurements of the ^{31}P NMR resonances of the principle storage components of the energy cycle,

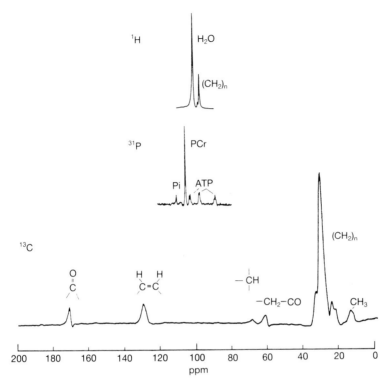

Fig. 9.1. High-resolution NMR spectra of human forearm tissue measured at 1.9 Tesla using a spectrometer developed by Oxford Research Systems. Upper trace, the proton spectrum; middle, ^{31}P; and lower, natural abundance carbon-13.

adenosine triphosphate and phosphocreatine. As can be seen in Fig. 9.1, these give clearly discernible resonances with data-acquisition times of a few minutes. Integration of the area beneath each resonance enables the amount of that species to be measured with an accuracy of 5–10 per cent.

From the standpoint of brain research, probably the most important results stem from the studies of neonates (Clady *et al.* 1983).

Unfortunately, the early successes with neonates did not lead to equivalent progress in adults. The relative intensities of the ^{31}P resonances of different chemical species were found to depend on the method used to excite the tissue. It is now known (Bottomley 1984) that this reflects the uncertainty of the spatial localization arising from the surface coil; responses are obtained from both the tissues of the scalp as well as those of the brain and depending on the subject studied, and the experimental conditions used, the relative contributions, and hence the composite spectrum, vary.

Although this was a technically predictable dénouement, in the context of this article it provides a convenient introduction to, and justification for, the remainder of this chapter which will be concerned with methods whereby spectra can be obtained from spatially defined volumes. As will be seen, most of these make use of the same linear field gradients as are used to produce tomographic images.

It will be recalled that the frequency at which a particular nuclear species gives a resonance is proportional to the field to which it is exposed. Advantage is taken of this fact in an imaging measurement to provide a spread of resonance frequencies which is spatially defined, by subjecting the object to a gradient of known magnitude and direction. This is illustrated in Fig. 9.2 with reference to the classical experiment of Lauterbur (1973). Application of a gradient in the Y-direction produces an NMR spectrum which shows the effective silhouette of the two tubes; when the gradient is in the X-direction the two silhouettes overlap.

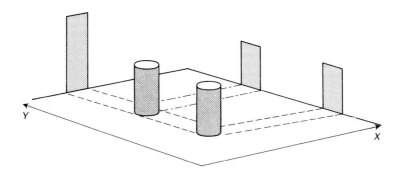

Fig. 9.2. Diagrammatic representation of the back-projection imaging method developed by Lauterbur. With a linear field gradient applied in the Y-direction, the NMR spectrum of two cylinders containing water shows as two separate projections. With the gradient along the X-axis the silhouettes of the two tubes coincide.

In both the above measurements the frequency bandwidth of the radio-frequency field used to excite the NMR responses was sufficiently wide to encompass the entire frequency spread produced by the field gradient. Clearly, if only a small, defined range of frequencies had been irradiated, it would have been possible to produce an image corresponding only to tube A (or to tube B). It is this combination of an applied gradient used to induce the spatially defined dispersion of resonance frequencies, along with frequency-selective excitation of specific resonance signals which is the basis for most of the methods discussed here.

Of course the procedure involving a single applied gradient actually defines a plane through the entire object. If a second gradient is applied at right angles to the first, then it will define an orthogonal plane; the interception between the two defines a line. Finally, if the third orthogonal gradient is applied, the common intercept between the three gradients defines a unique point. A variant on this concept provided the first versatile method for defining a volume anywhere within the object, known as the sensitive point method (Hinshaw 1976); it has more recently been extended. From the standpoint of point spectroscopy it suffers from several limitations, the principal of which is that it produces broadening of the resonances, which is undesirable (Scott *et al.* 1982) and we shall not again refer to it here.

The combined use of gradients and selective-excitation radiofrequency pulses is applicable to spectroscopic measurements made either with sur-face-coil or enclosed-volume probes. We shall discuss the former first. A sur-face coil produces a highly inhomogeneous distribution of radiofrequency field, in which the magnitude of the radiofrequency field falls off with increases in distance from the surface (Evelhoch and Ackerman 1983); this causes variations in the intensity of the resonance signal, even of a completely homogeneous object. Consider now the effect of applying a linear field gra-dient perpendicular to the surface of the coil; obviously this imposes a fre-quency spread in that direction. If a selective radiofrequency field is applied it will excite only a small section taken through the entire volume which is influ-enced by the surface coil; in effect, that volume will have been divided into a series of 'hockey-pucks', in each of which there is a reasonably homogeneous, vertical distribution of radiofrequency field (see Fig. 9.3). Of course the signal level will still vary from one level to the next so that absolute intensity comparisons between them will not be feasible without correction. Neverthe-less in this way it is trivial to distinguish between the signals from the surface of an object and those from deeper regions.

A very similar approach has been used by Haselgrove and co-workers (1983) with volume coils enclosing either a rat, or a gerbil; a slice thickness of ca. 4 mm was achieved for ^{31}P spectra.

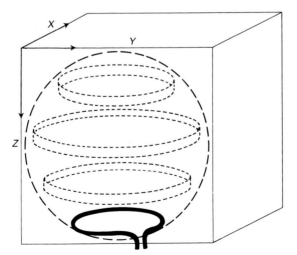

Fig. 9.3. Diagrammatic representation of the profile for radiofrequency penetration from a circular surface coil in the *x, y* plane. With a linear field gradient applied along the *Z*-direction it is possible to use a frequency-selective radiofrequency to obtain NMR signals from a specific slice at any depth in the sample.

Clinical studies in man at 1.5 Tesla have also been reported (Bottomley 1984). Advantage has been taken of the high spatial radiofrequency homogeneity of a whole-body-sized coil to irradiate the entire body; detection of the NMR signals using a surface coil then offers the advantage of increased filling-factor and hence S/N ratio, as compared with that of the longer coil. For ^{31}P spectra, 12 mm-thick slices were studied, and acceptable S/N ratios obtained in 5–20 min of time-averaging.

So far in this discussion we have emphasized methods which produce high-resolution spectra from a localized volume within the object. In the next section 'chemical-shift-resolved-tomography' will be explored, which produces separate images that display the spatial distribution of individual chemical species within a defined plane of known thickness. Several approaches have been suggested, and it has already been demonstrated that separate images can be obtained from water and fat in human tissues (Bottomley *et al.* 1984). As with the original proton tomography measurement, this topic was first explored by Lauterbur *et al.* (1975); subsequently, numerous other groups have also reported results (Cox and Styles 1980; Bottomley 1981; Brown *et al.* 1981; Hall and Sukumar 1982, 1984*b*; Maudsley *et al.* 1983; Mareci and Booker 1984).

The limiting experiment which is possible involves the generation of a four-dimensional data set which encodes in addition to the three spatial coordinates, the complete chemical shift range for each volume element. Once the data have been acquired, they can be interrogated in a variety of ways, two of which are illustrated in Fig. 9.4. Thus, a physical 'slice' can be defined in any direction and of any thickness and the spin density of each nuclear species within that volume which gives a resonance can then be viewed in projection on to that plane. (Figuratively this is equivalent to pulling one card from a pack of playing cards, and then splitting that card into separate slices, one corresponding to each colour.) Alternatively, the original data set can be re-evaluated to produce the composite spectrum corresponding to any arbitrary volume within the data space. The principal shortcoming of this particular class of measurement stems from the fact that each of the four dimensions has to be obtained separately. As a result the total data-acquisition time using conventional methods is prodigious; thus a $128 \times 128 \times 128 \times 128$ data set, with 1 s for each point, would take 24.3 days for acquisition, which is impractical. However, this is a rather misleading statistic and in practice useful data sets have already been obtained (Hall *et al.* 1984) in a few hours using standard procedures, and even that time can be reduced to a few tens of minutes with the use of fast-imaging methods (Mansfield and Pykett 1973; Hall and Sukumar 1984). Furthermore, measurements which have a modest reduction in dimensionality are even faster; an example of this is the three-dimensional imaging measurement (X, Y, δ) which encodes all the spectroscopic data (δ) from a particular plane (X, Y).

Some indication of the complexity of spectra which are amenable to this

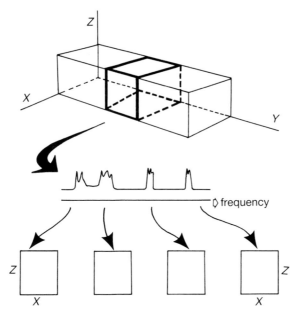

Fig. 9.4. Diagrammatic representation of the profile for radiofrequency penetration from a circular surface coil in the *x*, *y* plane. With a linear field gradient applied along the *Z*-direction it is possible to use a frequency-selective radiofrequency to obtain NMR signals from a specific slice at any depth in the sample.

type of experimentation is given in Fig. 9.5 (Hall and Sukumar 1984). The inset shows the composite spectrum of a series of organic molecules contained in 7 glass capillaries each 1 mm diameter and enclosed in a 5 mm diameter tube. The location of each tube was specified on the basis of the known magnitudes of the applied gradients, the spectrum of each tube was produced. It can be seen that additional peaks arise in some cases, but these can all be eliminated by an iterative computer procedure. The same original data set was also used to produce the slice images shown in Fig. 9.6. As can be seen, both the spatial- and the frequency-resolution images are excellent.

A further example of chemical shift resolution is given (Hall and Sukumar 1984*b*) in Fig. 9.7. In this case the data set was produced by a three-dimensional imaging method involving (X, Y) and (δ). The point of note is that each of the component lines of the ethanol spectrum could be separately processed to produce an image; given that these are separated by only ca. 7 Hz, this augurs well for the future of chemical shift resolved proton tomography.

Concern has been expressed that equivalent measurements will not be possible for heteronuclear species such as ^{31}P because of their low effective S/N ratio. Although that is certainly going to prevent many important measurements, it is premature to be totally negative. It will undoubtedly be

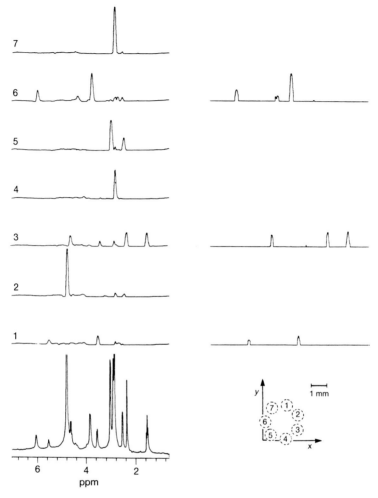

Fig. 9.5. Proton NMR measurements at 270 MHz of a phantom of seven glass capillaries (1 mm diameter) containing various organic liquids. The composite spectrum is shown in the lower trace. The spectra in the left hand column are derived by defining the spatial region corresponding to each tube. The equivalent traces in the right-hand column were obtained by a second iteration intended to eliminate the unwanted artifacts.

necessary to sacrifice some spatial resolution in the interests of time-saving. However, far greater savings will accrue from the use of fast-imaging methods. And even without either of those considerations, the total time required need not be excessive. For example, the total acquisition time required for the data set in Fig. 9.8 was only ca. 60 times longer than that for the equivalent proton image. Admittedly the phantom used was not an exacting one, yet the result is the first chemical-shift-resolved image based on [13]C

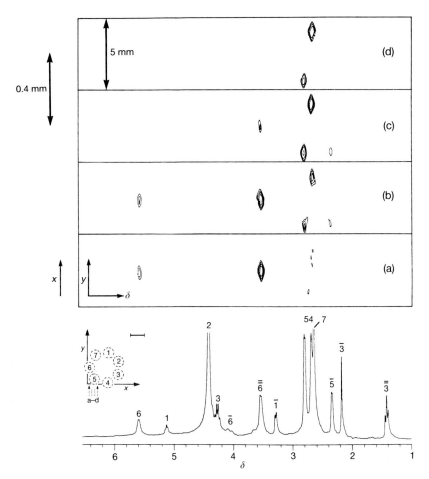

Fig. 9.6. Tomographic slice images derived from the same data set as the spectra in Fig. 9.5. The horizontal scale for traces a–d is identical to that of the composite spectra shown along the bottom. The superscript numbers correspond to the tube in which each substance is located. The region represented by each of the slices, a–d, is shown on the inset. Slice a shows principally the constituents in tube 6, and slice d those of tubes 5 and 7.

in natural abundance (Hall and Sukumar 1982). This too is a promising augury, especially if the approach were to make use of carbon-13-enriched substances to label specific metabolites.

Notwithstanding those opportunities, studies of proton spectra seem certain to provide a rapid entrée with brain biochemistry. The main technical difficulty stems from the proton resonance of the water in the tissues, which completely swamps the signals from species present in low concentration. Numerous methods are available whereby the water signal can be eliminated, and of these the most successful at present is the so-called '1:3:3:1 sequence'

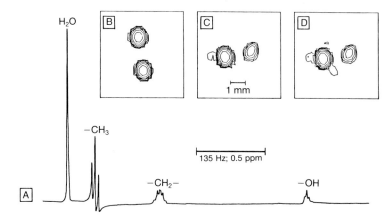

Fig. 9.7. Three-dimensional, chemical-shift-resolved tomography of a phantom of four tubes (1 mm diameter), two containing water and two ethanol. A separate image can be obtained for each separate line of the composite spectrum shown along the lower part.

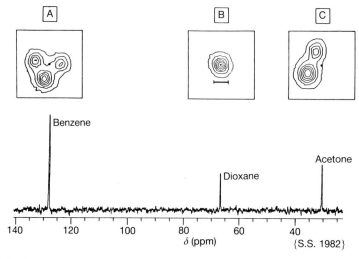

Fig. 9.8. Natural abundance carbon-13 chemical-shift-resolved tomograph of a series of capillaries containing organic liquids, measured using the Lauterbur method at 6.2 Tesla.

(Hore 1983). Using this, the proton resonances of many brain metabolites can be easily detected in a few minutes; and, as we have seen previously, the additional technology already exists for chemical-shift mapping.

Access to a device capable of combining all the spin physics of conventional NMR, along with control of three orthogonal linear field gradients opens up an immense array of new experiments. Rather than speculate about a wide range of these, here just two examples are mentioned which are under active study in this laboratory.

The first of these involves the *in vivo* measurement of self-diffusion coefficients, D, for molecules in human tissues. This parameter represents a measure of the random, Brownian motion in solution and hence provides, in principle at least, a time-weighted measure of the environments which a particular molecule encounters during its diffusion through the medium. Molecules in a more viscous medium will diffuse at a different rate from those in a less viscous one; similarly, in a given medium, a molecule which binds to bulky medium components, such as cell membranes or biopolymers, will have a different diffusion rate from one which has no such affinity. Measurements of the rates for water in various chemical environments have been reported for many years (Stejskal and Tanner 1965), and in the 1970s for excised animal tissues (Clark *et al.* 1982); the same basic method can be used for man. At the University of British Columbia this has been achieved (Hall and Luck, unpublished) using a surface coil, and the pulse sequence previously described by Stejskal and Tanner (1965). For human forearm muscle, separate signals were obtained for water and fat and the measured diffusion coefficients were, respectively, 1.7×10^{-9} m^{2}s^{-1} and 1.6×10^{-9} m^{2}s^{-1}. For water, the ratio was 0.57 which accords with the range of literature values (0.5–0.6) (Clark *et al.* 1982).

One of several technical limitations of NMR spectroscopy is that it demands that the magnet used provides a high field homogeneity over the entire volume of interest. This is never easy, and is always expensive; the current state-of-the-art is that a 1 m bore magnet provides 1 part in 10^7 homogeneity over a sphere of diameter ca. 14 cm, which is too small to encompass an adult head, let alone the torso. Short of a major breakthrough in magnet design, pursuit of spectroscopy in man requires a means for obtaining high-resolution spectra from larger volumes; remarkably, such a method exists. It has been known for some years (Kumar *et al.* 1975; Pouzard *et al.* 1981) that the linewidths of 'zero-quantum' transitions are independent of the homogeneity of the magnetic field to which the sample is exposed; this is in stark contrast to the situation for the single-quantum transitions which have been used exclusively up to the present time for all clinical magnetic-resonance studies.

It is not appropriate here to give the details of zero-quantum spectroscopy. Suffice it to say that methods have been developed (Hall and Norwood, unpublished) which enable zero-quantum spectra to be measured with reasonable efficiency in terms of 'signal-to-noise' per unit of time. An example from a chemical sample is given in Fig. 9.9 where it can be seen that when measured in an inhomogeneous field, the zero-quantum linewidths are comparable with those of the corresponding single-quantum spectra measured under optimal conditions. This approach will certainly not displace the need for conventional methods, yet it has some intriguing properties. For example, the fundamental transition selection rule for zero-quantum

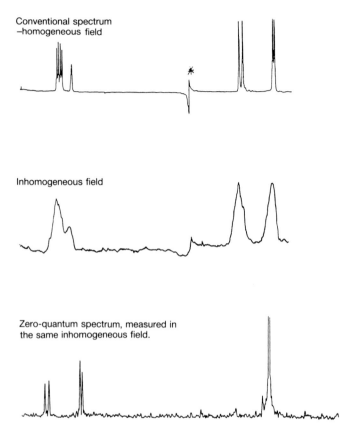

Fig. 9.9. Proton resonance spectra for vinyl acetate ($CH_2 = CHOCHCH_3$), measured at 270 MHz under conditions such that the methyl resonance is attenuated and folded over to give the peak indicated by *. The upper trace shows the conventional, single-quantum spectrum measured in a homogeneous magnetic field. The middle trace was measured under identical conditions, except that the homogeneity of the magnetic field had been intentionally degraded by mis-setting of the s in controls. The lower trace was measured in the same inhomogeneous field as the one above, but using a pulse sequence designed to give only the zero-quantum transitions; note that the transition frequencies are different for this trace.

NMR transitions is that the molecule have two or more inequivalent proton spins. This means that water, for example, cannot give a zero-quantum transition; thus, pulse imperfections apart, it is not necessary to develop special means to suppress the resonance of water; simply, a zero-quantum resonance cannot exist. It is also appropriate to note here that special pulse methods are also available which enable double, triple, and higher-quantum-level spectra to be elicited from molecules which have an appropriate number of inequivalent protons. These can be used as 'molecular filters' to reduce the number of molecules in a particular sample which can give rise to

NMR transitions, and hence be observed. However, it should be noted that the excitement that such prospects can raise must be tempered by the ever-present, and daunting, lack of signal-to-noise sensitivity, yet those with conventional proton tomographs need not fear that they will be excluded from these future opportunities since the requisite pulse sequences are not difficult to effect using any conventional imaging spectrometer.

In this final section, some of the clinical concepts which can be pursued using the technology mentioned earlier are assessed. The first of these involves attempts to distinguish normal from diseased tissue. For reasons which are not yet clearly known, the NMR properties of water in tissue provide an overall index for many pathological lesions of brain which can, as a result, be detected in a proton tomography image as regions which have heightened contrast. For example (Young *et al.* 1981), many tumours, multiple sclerosis plaques, regions of ischaemia, or haemorrhage are clearly visible in images which have been contrasted on the basis of differentials in either the spin–spin, or the spin–lattice, relaxation times. This clearly illustrates the subtle molecular interactions which govern the properties of water in mammalian tissue; at present, very little is known about the molecular basis for these observations.

It now remains to establish whether or not additional insight can be obtained via NMR spectroscopic measurements, for example, whether distinctions can be made between benign and malignant tumours as was originally suggested by Damadian (1971). An efficient protocol for such measurements would be to use conventional proton tomography to provide a three-dimensional anatomical map of the brain and, possibly, to identify the regions of interest. The resultant spatial coordinates would then enable the spectrometer to be 'tuned' to those regions to provide the appropriate spectra. Using existing technology such an evaluation could be achieved without need to reposition the patient. Furthermore, it is possible to measure the resonance signals from more than one nuclear species so the spectroscopic measurements need not be confined to protons.

If the particular study were to involve a series of spectroscopic measurements across a large volume of brain (as distinct from a few, small locations) then it might be more efficient to perform a chemical-shift-resolve imaging measurement of the entire head.

Difficult as they are, such distinctions of gross pathology are still easier than detection of neuropsychiatric phenomena or of subtle biochemical lesions, especially those which take place at the receptor level. Such measurements will require extremely subtle methodology, and even then may not be viable; nevertheless, with ingenuity, seemingly impossible measurements can be made. One example will suffice to illustrate this point. Consider the detection of a small quantity of copper, 2μ, say (25×10^{-6} g). *Direct* detection by NMR means is completely impossible. However, copper ions are paramagnetic and as a result influence the relaxation rate of water molecules with which they make contact. Given the free exchange of water molecules between those in the primary solvation shell and those in the bulk solvent, it follows that one copper ion can sufficiently influence the relaxation properties of a large enough number of water molecules for this effect to be easily detected in an imaging (or spectroscopic) measurement (Hall and Rajanayagam, unpublished). This is an example of the concept of 'molecular-amplification' in which the information of interest cannot be *directly* detected but can be transferred to a reporter group which is present in higher abundance. It and other concepts which combine the skills of the NMR-spectroscopic and synthetic chemist will, if guided by the appropriate questions, play pivotal rôles as we seek to determine not only how the brain functions, but how dysfunction can be detected, treated, and corrected.

ACKNOWLEDGEMENTS

It is a pleasure to thank numerous friends and colleagues both in Canada and the UK for stimulating discussions, and especially my graduate students. The work from the University of British Columbia was supported by the Natural Sciences and Engineering Research Council of Canada and the Medical Research Council of Canada.

REFERENCES

Ackerman, J. J. H., Grove, T. H., Wong, G. C., Cadian, D. G., and Radda, G. K. (1980). Mapping of metabolites in whole animals by ^{31}P Nuclear Magnetic Resonance using surface coils. *Nature, Lond.* **283** , 167–70.

Bendel, P., Lai, C.-M., and Lauterbur, P. C. (1980). ^{31}P Spectroscopic Zeugmatography of phosphorous metabolites. *J. Magn. Reson.* **38** , 343–56.

Bottomley, P. A. (1981). A versatile magnetic field gradient control system for NMR imaging. *J. Phys. E.* **14** , 1081–7.

—— (1984). Paper presented at the British Radiofrequency Spectroscopy Group Meeting, University of Surrey, U.K., September 19–21.

—— Hart, H. R., Edelstein, W. A., Schenk, J. F., Smith, L. S., Leve, W. M., Mueller, D. M., and Redington, R. W. (1984). Anatomy and metabolism of the normal human brain studied by magnetic resonance at 1.5 Tesla. *Radiology* **150** , 441–6.

Brown, T. R., Kincaid, B. M., and Uguril, K. (1981). Nuclear magnetic resonance shift imaging in three dimensions. *Proc. Natl. Acad. Sci., U.S.A.* **79** , 3523–6.

Caldy, E. B., de L. Costello, A. M., Dawson, M. J., Delpy, D. T., Hope, P. L., Reynolds, E. O. R., Tofts, P. S., and Wilkie, D. R. (1983). Non-invasive investigation of cerebral metabolism in newborn infants by phosphorous nuclear magnetic resonance spectroscopy. *Lancet* **i** , 1059–2.

Clark, M. E., Burnell, E. E., Chapman, N. R., and Hinke, J. A. M. (1982). Water in barnacle muscle. IV. Factors contributing to reduced self-diffusion. *Biophys. J.* **39** , 289–99.

Cox, S. J. and Styles, P. (1980). Towards biochemical imaging. *J. Magn. Reson.* **40** , 209–12.

Damadian, R. (1971). Tumor detection by nuclear magnetic resonance. *Science* **171** 1151–3.

Evelhoch, J. L. and Ackerman, J. J. H. (1983). NMR T_1 measurements in Inhomogenous B_1 with surface coils. *J. Magn. Reson.* **53** , 52–64.

Gordon, R. E., Hanley, P. E., Shaw, D., Gadian, D. G., Radda, G. K., Styles, P., Bore, P. J., and Chan, L. (1980). Location of metabolites in animals using ^{31}P topical magnetic resonance. *Nature, Lond.* **287** , 736–8.

Hall, L. D. and Sukumar, S. (1982). Chemical microscopy using a high resolution nuclear magnetic resonance spectrometer. A combination of tomography/spectroscopy using either proton or carbon-13. *J. Magn. Reson.* **50**, 161–4.

—— and —— (1984*a*). Rapid data-acquisition technique for NMR imaging by the projection-construction method. *J. Magn. Reson.* **56**, 179–82.

—— and —— (1984*b*). Three-dimensional Fourier transform NMR imaging. High resolution chemical-shift-resolved planar imaging. *J. Magn. Reson.* **56**, 314–17.

—— and —— 1984*c*). A new image-processing method for NMR chemical microscopy. *J. Magn. Reson.* **56**, 326–33.

—— Rayajayagam, V. and Sukamar, S. (1985). *J. Magn. Reson.* (in press).

Haselgrove, J. C., Subramaniam, V. H., Leigh, J. S., Guylai, L., and Chance, B. (1983). *In vivo* one-dimensional imagery of phosphorous-31 nuclear magnetic resonance. *Science* **220**, 1170–3.

Hinshaw, W. S. (1976). Image formation by nuclear magnetic resonance: The sensitive point method. *J. Appl. Phys.* **47**, 3709–21.

Hore, P. J. (1983). A new method for water suppression in the proton NMR spectra of aqueous solutions. *J. Magn. Reson.* **54** 539–42.

Kumar, A., Welti, D. I., and Ernst, R. R. (1975). Fourier Zeugmatography. *J. Magn. Reson.* **18**, 69–83.

Lauterbur, P. C. (1973). Image formation by induced local interactions; examples employing nuclear magnetic resonance. *Nature, Lond.* **242**, 190–1.

—— Kramer, D. M., House, W. V., and Chen, C. N. (1975). Zeugmatographic high resolution nuclear magnetic resonance spectroscopy. Images of clinical inhomogeneity within macroscopic objects. *J. Amer. Chem. Soc.* **97**, 6866–68.

Mansfield, P. and Pykett, I. L. (1978). Biological and chemical imaging by NMR. *J. Magn. Reson.* **29**, 355–73.

Mareci, T. H. and Booker, H. R. (1984). High resolution magnetic resonance spectra from a sensitive region defined with pulsed field gradients. *J. Magn. Reson.* **57**, 157–63.

Maudsley, A. A., Hilal, S. K., Perman, W. H., and Simon, H. E. (1983). Spatially Resolved High Resolution Spectroscopy by Four-Dimensional NMR. *J. Magn. Reson.* **51**, 147–52.

Pouzard, G., Hall, L. D., and Sukumar, S. (1981). High resolution, zero quantum transition (two-dimensional) nuclear magnetic resonance spectroscopy: spectral analysis. *J. Amer. Chem. Soc.* **103**, 4209–15.

Ross, B. D., Radda, G. K., Rocker, G., Esiri, M., and Falconer, J. (1981). Examination of a case of suspected McArdle's syndrome by [31]P Nuclear Magnetic Resonance. *N. Engl. J. Med.* **304**, 1338–42.

Scott, K. N., Brooker, H. R., Fitzsimmons, J. R., Bennett, H. F., and Mick, R. C. (1982). Spatial localization of ^{31}P nuclear magnetic resonance signal by the sensitive point method. *J. Magn. Reson.* **50**, 339–44.

Stejskal, E. O. and Tanner, J. E. (1965). Spin diffusion measurements: Spin echoes in the presence of a time-dependent field gradient. *J. Chem. Phys.* **42**, 288–92.

Young, I. R., Hall, A. S., Pallis, C. A., Bydder, G. M., Legg, N. J., and Steiner, R. E. (1981). Nuclear magnetic resonance imaging of the brain in multiple sclerosis. *Lancet* **ii**, 1063–6.

—— Bailes, D. R., Burl, M., Collins, A. G., Smith, D. T., MacDonnell, M. J., Orr, J. S., Banks, L. M., Bydder, G. M., Greenspan, R. H., and Steiner, R. E. (1982). Initial clinical evaluation of a whole body nuclear magnetic resonance (NMR) tomograph. *J. Comput. Assist. Tomogr.* **6**, 1–18.

10

Nuclear magnetic resonance studies and the potential of this technique for use in psychiatry

EVE C. JOHNSTONE, G. M. BYDDER, T. J. CROW, D. G. C. OWENS, AND R. E. STEINER

INTRODUCTION

When the nuclei of certain atoms are placed in a magnetic field they can be made to absorb or emit electromagnetic radiation. The observation of this phenomenon—nuclear magnetic resonance or NMR—was first reported in 1946 by the groups of Bloch and Purcell. The spectrum of absorbed or emitted electromagnetic radiation depends upon the nature of the nucleus of interest and its local chemical environment. Only nuclei with an odd number of protons or neutrons are NMR-responsive and this of course restricts its possibilities. The available nuclei of biological interest include hydrogen nuclei (protons), phosphorus, sodium, and carbon. Of the nuclei responsive to NMR, hydrogen nuclei (each of which consists of a single proton) are by far the most abundant in the human body in the form of protons in water. While ^{23}Na and ^{31}P imaging have been shown to be feasible, in general, clinical imaging as it is so far developed concerns hydrogen nuclei. The first published NMR image was produced by Lauterbur in 1973 and during the 1970s groups in the UK (Andrew 1980; Holland et al. 1980; Hounsfield 1980; Mallard 1981; Ordidge et al. 1981) and the USA (Crooks et al. 1982; Ross et al. 1982) developed proton-imaging systems, and clinical trials began about 1980. Experience has so far been limited to about 8000 patients worldwide.

PRINCIPLES OF THE TECHNIQUE

All NMR machines are constructed around a large magnet which produces a uniform static magnetic field. In the absence of any externally applied magnetic field, hydrogen nuclei or protons are randomly positioned but they behave like little bar magnets. In the presence of the static magnetic field produced by the magnet in the NMR machine the protons line up in the direction of the field producing a net nuclear magnetization in the long axis of the patient. Additional radiofrequency (RF) magnetic pulses are applied by means of a coil which surrounds the patient (Fig. 10.1). These pulses are used to rotate the nuclear magnetization after which it returns to its original

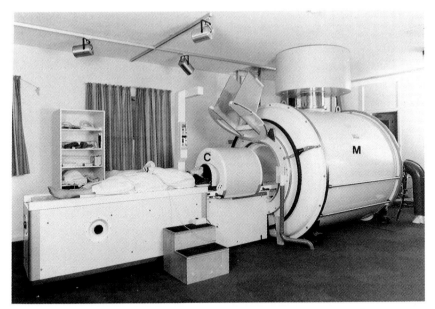

Fig. 10.1. An NMR imaging machine. M, the magnet; C, the receiver coil.

position. For example, if a 90° pulse is applied the nuclear magnetization is rotated from the longitudinal direction into the transverse plane. Following this rotation the component of the magnetization in the long axis of the patient recovers from zero to its original amplitude in an exponential way. This recovery is called longitudinal or spin-lattice relaxation and is characterized by the time constant T_1.

Relaxation of the component of the magnetization in the transverse direction back to its original amplitude of zero is termed transverse or spin–spin relaxation and is characterized by time constant T_2. A receiver coil surrounds the patient and the changing magnetization induces an electrical signal in this coil. The signal after a 90° pulse is known as the free induction decay (FID).

Longitudinal relaxation (T_1) depends on the interaction of protons with surrounding nuclei and molecules (the 'lattice') while transverse relaxation (T_2) depends on the interaction of protons with each other. Both T_1 and T_2 are sensitive indices of the local nuclear and molecular environment. By using a variety of pulse sequences it is possible to produce images with varying dependence on proton density p, T_1, and T_2. Several commonly used pulse sequences designed to do this are shown in Table 10.1.

HAZARDS OF NMR

No adverse effects of NMR have been reported, although some theoretical risks of the procedure, most of which relate to overheating, have been

TABLE 10.1. *Commonly used pulse sequences.*

Pulse sequences	Principal image parameters
Free induction decay (FID)	Proton density
Inversion-recovery (IR)	T_1 proton density
Spin-echo (SE)	T_2 proton density

described and are discussed by Budinger (1981). The only known potential serious hazard of practical relevance at the present time is the possiblity that ferromagnetic aneurysm clips might be dislodged by the magnetic fields (New *et al.* 1983) and patients with these *in situ* should not be examined. The procedure does involve the patients being enclosed in a narrow metal tube where his attendants cannot really see him and cannot touch him. The duration of the examination is variable depending upon the number of sites to be studied but is usually over a hour. About 5 per cent of patients become so anxious in this situation that the procedure has to be abandoned. This figure might be higher if a less gravely ill population than that which has generally so far been examined were considered.

USEFULNESS OF NMR

The main focus of clinical interest with NMR has been the brain although imaging of other organs is providing useful clinical information. It is possible to obtain a high degree of contrast between grey and white matter and this displays considerable anatomical detail which is not defined with computed tomography. The posterior fossa can be visualized much better than with X-ray CT scans because there is no bone artefact and sagittal and coronal images are readily obtained (Fig. 10.2).

Vascular disease

Cerebral infarction produces a loss of grey–white matter contrast on inversion recovery scans and NMR is particularly useful for demonstration of brain stem infarcts because of the absence of bone artefact. Intracerebral and subdural haemorrhages are both readily visualized.

Infection

Abscesses have been well shown with inversion recovery and spin-echo scans although calcification is poorly visualized. Herpes encephalitis is associated with regions of prolonged T_1 and T_2 values and may give a strikingly abnormal picture. Because of the absence of bone artefact the temporal lobes, which are a relatively frequent site of this disease, are well shown.

Demyelinating disease

The high level of grey–white matter contrast seen with inversion recovery scans provides a basis for the application of NMR to demyelinating disease.

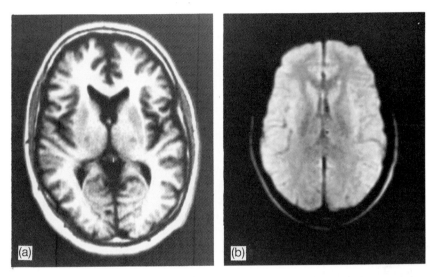

Fig. 10.2. (a) A normal inversion-recovery (T_1) scan (b) a normal spin-echo (T_2) scan.

In an initial study of ten patients with multiple sclerosis, Young *et al.* (1981) found many more lesions with NMR than with CT. Since then the value of NMR in demonstrating the lesions of multiple sclerosis has been shown repeatedly and rare disorders of white matter such as radiation damage and Binswanger's disease can also be demonstrated (Fig. 10.3).

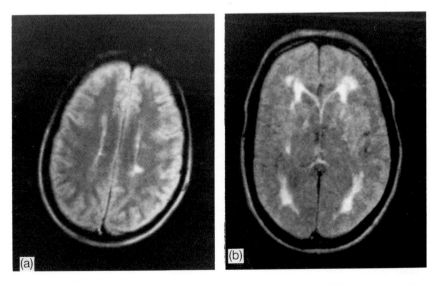

Fig. 10.3. (a) NMR scan of multiple sclerosis (M.S.); (b) an NMR scan of multiple infarction.

Hydrocephalus

The ventricular system is well visualized in NMR as it is in CT. NMR offers the advantage of showing periventricular oedema on spin-echo scans and this may be of value in the recognition of acute ventricular shunt problems.

Tumours

These are well demonstrated, and the lack of bone artefact is a significant advantage in posterior fossa lesions. It may be difficult with NMR to differentiate the tumour edge from the surrounding oedema. In some cases this is more clearly defined with contrast enhanced CT scans. Paramagnetic contrast agents have however now been developed for use with NMR and may be valuable in this context (Fig. 10.4).

Relevance of NMR to psychiatry

It is clear that NMR is likely to have a place in the investigation of organic psychiatric disorders but its role outside of this area is at present unknown. A study of the NMR appearances in schizophrenia has been conducted using patients from Northwick Park Hospital and the NMR scanner at the Hammersmith Hospital. The reduction in brain substance, implied by the increased lateral ventricular size found in some schizophrenic patients (Johnstone *et al.* 1976; Owens *et al.* 1985), has been confirmed by a *post mortem* study (Brown *et al.* 1985). The cause of this cell loss or shrinkage is unknown, but it is possible that it might result from a pathological process associated with periventricular swelling or inflammation in the acute phase. In order to examine this hypothesis, the periventricular appearances of four groups of young schizophrenic patients were compared with those of age-matched controls (Table 10.2).

TABLE 10.2. *Groups of schizophrenic patients in the NMR study described in the text.*

Group	Number and sex distribution	Age
Poor outcome never normal	6 M	23.3 ± 3.3
Poor outcome once normal	4 M	22.7 ± 3.5
Good outcome once normal	6 M	23.0 ± 2.1
Neuroleptic-free 1st episode	10 M; 1 F	21.8 ± 3.6
Normal controls	12 M	24.7 ± 3

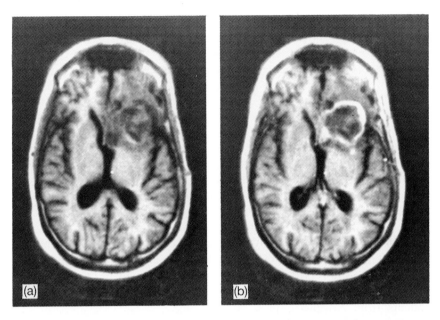

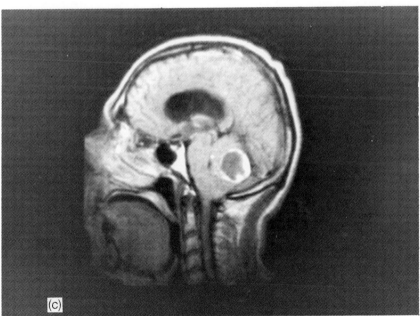

Fig. 10.4. (a) NMR scan of an astrocytoma Grade IV. (b) an enhanced NMR scan of the tumour shown in (a). (c) an enhanced NMR scan of a metastasis from the breast (sagittal view).

The principal comparison was between normal controls and patients with untreated first schizophrenic episodes. If differences were found it would be important to know if the abnormalities persisted beyond the first episode and whether or not such persistence was associated with the nature of the outcome of the episode. Patients with varying degrees of recovery from first schizophrenic episodes were therefore selected for NMR from the participants of a recently completed large study of first-episode schizophrenia (Macmillan *et al.* 1985). The scans were reviewed by the radiologists involved who considered that some spin-echo films showed an unusual increase in the light area at the anterolateral angles of the ventricles. They demonstrated this and the normal appearance of this area to the clinicians involved, and all five investigators blindly rated the appearances in every subject as normal, possibly with increased light area and definitely with increased light area. The inter-rater reliability was high (Kendal's $W = 0.53$; $P \pm 0.00001$) and no individual rater deviated significantly from the remainder. Ratings from all investigators were therefore summed and the cases were ranked in terms of this figure. The results were as follows (Fig. 10.5). There were no significant differences between any of the groups and

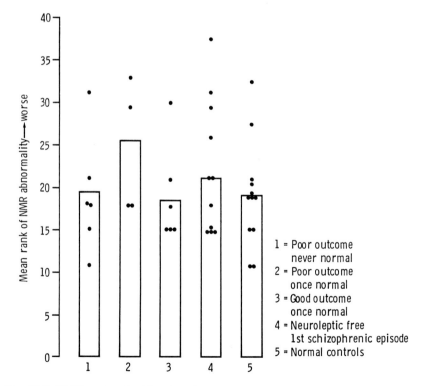

Fig. 10.5. NMR scans of schizophrenics and normal controls in terms of putative abnormality.

no difference between all schizophrenics and controls. Some individuals with a high rank in terms of numbers of investigators rating them as definitely abnormal were found in all groups including the control sample. The results indicated that the appearance of an increased light area at the anterolateral angles of the ventricles is not related to the nature of an early schizophrenic episode or indeed to the diagnosis of schizophrenia.

Constant improvements in the resolution of NMR images are now in progress. In using an advancing technique one is in the position that the method used in any investigation may well be obsolete by the time the study has been completed. Some of our latest scans in schizophrenic patients show appearances which may be abnormal but the range of appearances in the normal population is unknown. Because of the rapid development of this area of technology repeated studies involving the blind assessment of patients and controls are likely to be required. This technique does, however, provide firm diagnostic evidence in disorders like multiple sclerosis where formerly the course of illness over years was often the best guide to diagnosis. This same criterion remains one of the best guides to diagnosis in functional psychotic illness but it is possible that developments of the technique of NMR may yet provide the concrete diagnostic evidence that has so long been sought.

REFERENCES

Andrew, E. R. (1980). NMR imaging of intact biological systems. *Phil. Trans Roy. Soc. Lond. (Biol.)* **289**, 471–81.

Bloch, F., Hansen, W. W., and Packard, M. E. (1946). Nuclear induction. *Phys. Rev.* **70**, 460–73.

Brown, R., Colter, N., Corsellis, N. A. N., Crow, T. J., Frith, C. D., Jagoe, R., Johnstone, E. C., and Marsh, L. (1985). Brain weight and parahippocampal cortical width are decreased and temporal horn is increased in schizophrenia in comparison with affective disorder. *Arch. Gen. Psychiat.* (in press).

Budinger, T. F. (1981). Nuclear magnetic resonance (NMR) *in vivo* studies: known thresholds for health effects. *J. Comp. Assist. Tomogr.* **5**, 800–11.

Crooks, L. E., Arakawa, M., Hoenninger, J., Watts, J., McRee, R., Kaufman, L., Davis, P. L., Margulis, A. R., and DeGroot, J. (1982). Nuclear magnetic resonance whole-body imager operating at 3.5 K Gauss. *Radiology* **143**, 169–74.

Holland, G. N., Moore, W. S., and Hawkes, R. C. (1980). Nuclear magnetic resonance tomography of the brain. *J. Comput. Assist. Tomogr.* **4**, 1–3.

Hounsfield, G. N. (1980). Computer medical imaging. *J. Comput. Assist. Tomogr.* **4**, 665–74.

Johnstone, E. C., Crow, T. J., Frith, C. D., Husband, J., and Kreel, L. (1976). Cerebral ventricular size and cognitive impairment in chronic schizophrenia. *Lancet* **ii**, 924–6.

Lauterbur, P. C. (1973). Image formation by induced local interactions: examples employing NMR. *Nature, Lond.* **242**, 190–1.

Macmillan, J. F., Crow, T. J., Johnson, A. L., and Johnstone, E. C. (1985). The Northwick Park study of first episodes of schizophrenia, 3, the short-term outcome. *Br. J. Psychiat.* (in press).

Mallard, J. (1981). The noes have it! Do they? *Brit. J. Radiol.* **54**, 831–49.

New, P. F. J., Rosen, B. R., Brady, T. J., Buonanno, F. S., Kistler, J. P., Burt, C. T.,

Hinshaw, W. S., Newhouse, J. H., Pohost, G. M., and Taveras, J. M. (1983). Potential hazards and artefacts of ferromagnetic and non-ferromagnetic surgical and dental materials and devices in nuclear magnetic resonance imaging. *Raldiology* **147**, 139–48.

Ordidge, R. J., Mansfield, P., and Coupland, R. E. (1981). Rapid biomedical imaging by NMR. *Brit. J. Radiol.* **54**, 850–5.

Owens, D. G. C., Johnstone, E. C., Crow, T. J., Frith, C. D., Jagoe, J. R., and Kreel, L. (1985). Lateral ventricular size in schizophrenia: relationship to the disease process and its clinical manifestations. *Psychol. Med.* **15**, 27–41.

Purcell, E. M., Torrey, H. C., and Pound, R. V. (1946). Resonance absorption by nuclear magnetic movements in a solid. *Phys. Rev.* **69**, 37.

Ross, R. J., Thompson, J. S., Kim, K., and Bailey, R. R. (1982). Nuclear magnetic resonance imaging and evaluation of human breast tissue: preliminary clinical trials. *Radiology* **143**, 195–205.

Young, I. R., Hall, A. S., Pallis, C. A., Legg, N. J., Bydder, G. M., and Steiner, R. E. (1981). Nuclear magnetic resonance imaging of the brain in multiple sclerosis. *Lancet.* **ii**, 1063–6.

Index